THE AFFORDA␣ FRYER COOｋ␣␣␣␣␣

Table of Contents

Air Fryer and Keto

Series 2

By Marisa Smith and Jason Smith

 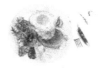

KETO DIET FOR WOMEN OVER 50

Contents

Chapter 4: Top 20 Keto Recipes 189

The Affordable Air Fryer Cookbook

The Ultimate Guide with 100 Quick and Delicious Affordable Recipes for beginners

By Marisa Smith

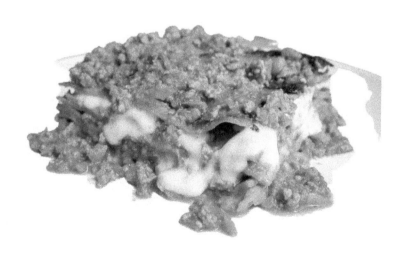

Introduction

We all love the deep-fried food taste, but not the calories or hassle of frying in too much fat. To solve this issue, the Air fryer was designed as its revolutionary nature allows you to cook food while frying with one or two tablespoons of oil and remove extra fat from the meal. This recipe book includes some of the amazing recipes that your Air fryer can prepare. From French fries to spring rolls and even soufflés, the choices are limitless!

Air Fryer Recipes

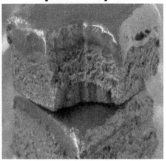

1. Chewy Breakfast Brownies

Total time: 40 min

Prep time: 10 min

Cook time: 30 min

Yield: 9 servings

Ingredients:

- 1 egg
- 2 tbsp. cocoa powder
- 1 tsp. vanilla
- 1 1/4 cup milk
- 1/2 cup applesauce
- 1/4 cup brown sugar
- 2 1/4 cup quick oats

Directions:

1. Spray and set aside a 9*9-inch baking dish with cooking spray.

2. Insert a rack of wire in rack position 6. Pick bake, set temperature to 350 f, 30-minute timer. To preheat the oven, press start.

3. Mix brown sugar, cocoa powder, and oats together in a big cup.

4. Add wet ingredients: blend until well mixed.

5. Pour the baking dish with the mixture and spread it properly.

6. Place foil on the baking dish and bake for 15 minutes. After 15 minutes, remove the cover and bake for 15 more minutes.

7. Enjoy and serve.

2.Peach Banana Baked Oatmeal

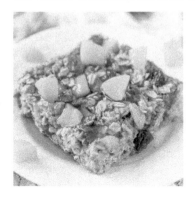

Total time: 45 min

Prep time: 10 min

Cook time: 35 min

Yield: 5 servings

Ingredients:

- Two eggs
- 1 tsp. vanilla
- 1 1/2 cups milk
- 1/2 tsp. cinnamon
- 3/4 tsp. baking powder
- 1/4 cup ground flax seed
- 2 1/2 cups steel-cut oats
- 2 bananas, sliced
- 1 peach, sliced
- 1/2 tsp. salt

Directions:

1. Spray an 8*8-inch baking dish with cooking spray and set aside.

2. Insert wire rack in rack position 6. Select bake, set temperature 350 f, timer for 35 minutes. Press start to preheat the oven.

3. Add all ingredients except one banana into the mixing bowl and mix until well combined.

4. Pour mixture into the baking dish and spread well. Spread the remaining 1 banana slices on top and bake for 35 minutes.

5. Serv e and enjoy.

3.Healthy Poppy seed Baked Oatmeal

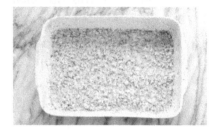

Total time: 35 min

Prep time: 10 min

Cook time: 25 min

Yield: 8 servings

Ingredients:

- 3 eggs
- 1 tbsp. poppy seeds
- 1 tsp. baking powder
- 1 tsp. vanilla
- 1 tsp. lemon zest
- 1/4 cup lemon juice
- 1/4 cup honey
- 2 cups almond milk
- 3 cups rolled oats
- 1/4 tsp. salt

Directions:

1. Spray a baking dish with cooking spray and set it aside.
2. Insert wire rack in rack position 6. Select bake, set temperature 350 f, timer for 25 minutes. Press start to preheat the oven.

3. In a large bowl, mix together all ingredients: until well combined.

4. Pour mixture into the baking dish and spread well, and bake for 25 minutes.

5. Serve and enjoy.

4.Healthy Berry Baked Oatmeal

Total time: 30 min

Prep time: 10 min

Cook time: 20 min

Yield: 4 servings

Ingredients:

- 1 egg
- 1 cup blueberries
- 1/2 cup blackberries
- 1/2 cup strawberries, sliced
- 1/4 cup maple syrup
- 1 1/2 cups milk
- 1 1/2 tsp. baking powder
- 2 cups old fashioned oats
- 1/2 tsp. salt

Directions:

1. Spray with cooking spray on a baking dish and put aside.

2. Insert a rack of wire in rack position 6. Pick bake, set temperature to 375 f, 20 minute timer. To preheat the oven, press start.

3. Blend together the peas, salt and baking powder in a mixing cup. Stir well and Mix vanilla, egg, maple syrup, and tea.

4. Add berries and blend well with them. Into the baking bowl, add the mixture and bake for 20 minutes.

5. Enjoy and serve.

5.Apple Oatmeal Bars

Total time: 35 min

Prep time: 10 min

Cook time: 25 min

Yield: 12 servings

Ingredients:

- 2 eggs
- 2 tbsp. butter
- 2 tsp. baking powder
- 2 cups apple, chopped
- 3 cups old fashioned oats
- Pinch of salt
- 1/2 cup honey
- 1 tbsp. vanilla
- 1 cup milk
- 1 tbsp. cinnamon

Directions:

1. Spray a 9*13-inch baking dish with cooking spray and set aside.
2. Insert wire rack in rack position 6. Select bake, set temperature 375 f, timer for 25 minutes. Press start to preheat the oven.
3. In a mixing bowl, mix together dry ingredients.
4. In a separate bowl, whisk together wet ingredients. Pour wet ingredient mixture into the dry mixture and mix well.
5. Pour mixture into the baking dish and bake for 25 minutes.
6. Slice and serve.

6.Walnut Banana Bread

Prep time: 10 minutes

Cook time: 50 minutes

Yield: 10 servings

Ingredients:

- 3 eggs
- 1 tsp. baking soda
- 4 tbsp. olive oil
- 1/2 cup walnuts, chopped
- 2 cups almond flour
- 3 bananas

Directions:

1. Grease loaf pan with butter and set aside.
2. Insert wire rack in rack position 6. Select bake, set temperature 350 f, timer for 50 minutes. Press start to preheat the oven.
3. Add all ingredients into the food processor and process until combined.
4. Pour batter into the prepared loaf pan and bake for 50 minutes.
5. Slices and serve.

7.Cinnamon Zucchini Bread

Total time: 1 hour 10 min

Prep time: 10 min

Cook time: 60 min

Yield: 12 servings

Ingredients:

- 3 eggs
- 1/2 tsp. nutmeg
- 1 1/2 tsp. baking powder

- 1 1/2 tsp. erythritol
- 2 1/2 cups almond flour
- 1 tsp. vanilla
- 1/2 cup walnuts, chopped
- 1 cup zucchini, grated & squeeze out all liquid
- 1/4 tsp. ground ginger
- 1 tsp. cinnamon
- 1/2 cup olive oil
- 1/2 tsp. salt

Directions:

1. Grease loaf pan with butter and set aside.
2. Insert wire rack in rack position 6. Select bake, set temperature 350 f, timer for 60 minutes. Press start to preheat the oven.
3. In a bowl, whisk eggs, vanilla, and oil. Set aside.
4. In a separate bowl, mix together almond flour, ginger, cinnamon, nutmeg, baking powder, salt, and sweetener. Set aside.
5. Add grated zucchini into the egg mixture and stir well.
6. Add dry ingredients into the egg mixture and stir to combine.
7. Pour batter into the loaf pan and bake for 60 minutes.
8. Slices and serve.

8. Italian Breakfast Bread

Total time: 60 min

Prep time: 10 min

Cook time: 50 min

Yield: 10 servings

Ingredients:

- 1/2 cup black olives, chopped
- 5 sun-dried tomatoes, chopped
- 2 tbsp. psyllium husk powder
- 5 egg whites
- 2 egg yolks
- 4 tbsp. coconut oil
- 2 cups flaxseed flour
- 2 tbsp. apple cider vinegar
- 1 tbsp. thyme, dried
- 1 tbsp. oregano, dried
- 2 1/2 oz. feta cheese
- 1 tbsp. baking powder
- 1/2 cup boiling water
- 1/2 tsp. salt

Directions:

1. Grease loaf pan with butter and set aside.
2. Insert wire rack in rack position 6. Select bake, set temperature 350 f, timer for 50 minutes. Press start to preheat the oven.
3. In a bowl, mix together psyllium husk powder, baking powder, and flaxseed.
4. Add oil and eggs and stir to combine. Add vinegar and stir well.
5. Add boiling water and stir to combine.
6. Add tomatoes, olives, and feta cheese. Mix well.
7. Pour batter into the loaf pan and bake for 50 minutes.
8. Sliced and serve.

9.Coconut Zucchini Bread

Total time: 55 min

Prep time: 10 min

Cook time: 45 min

Yield: 12 servings

Ingredients:

- 1 banana, mashed
- 1 tsp. stevia
- 4 eggs
- 1/2 cup coconut flour
- 1 tbsp. coconut oil
- 1 cup zucchini, shredded and squeeze out all liquid
- 1/2 cup walnuts, chopped
- 1 tbsp. cinnamon
- 3/4 tsp. baking soda
- 1/2 tsp. salt
- 1 tsp. apple cider vinegar
- 1/2 tsp. nutmeg

Directions:

1. Grease the loaf pan and set it aside with butter.
2. Wire rack insertion at rack position 6. Pick bake, set temperature to 350 f, 45 minute timer. To preheat the oven, press start.
3. Whisk the egg, banana, oil and stevia together in a big mug.
4. Stir well and add all the dried ingredients, vinegar, and zucchini. Combine the walnuts and stir.
5. Through the loaf tin, add the batter and bake for 45 minutes.
6. Slicing and cooking.

10. Protein Banana Bread

Total time: 1 hour 20 min

Prep time: 10 min

Cook time: 1 hour 10 min

Yield: 16 servings

Ingredients:

- 3 eggs
- 1/3 cup coconut flour
- 1/2 cup swerve
- 2 cups almond flour
- 1/2 cup ground chia seed
- 1/2 tsp. vanilla extract
- 4 tbsp. butter, melted
- 3/4 cup almond milk
- 1 tbsp. baking powder
- 1/3 cup protein powder
- 1/2 cup water
- 1/2 tsp. salt

Directions:

1. Grease the loaf pan and set it aside with butter.
2. Wire rack insertion at rack position 6. Bake selection, set temperature 325 f, 1 hour 10 minutes timer. To preheat the oven, press start.
3. Whisk the chia seed and 1/2 cup of water together in a small dish. Only put aside.
4. Mix the almond flour, baking powder, protein powder, coconut flour, sweetener, and salt together in a big cup.
5. Mix eggs, sugar, blend of chia seeds, vanilla extract and butter until well mixed.
6. In the prepared loaf tin, add the batter and bake for 1 hour and 10 minutes.

7. Slicing and serving

11. Easy Kale Muffins

Total time: 40 min

Prep time: 10 min

Cook time: 30 min

Yield: 8 servings

Ingredients:

- 6 eggs
- 1/2 cup milk
- 1/4 cup chives, chopped
- 1 cup kale, chopped
- Pepper
- Salt

Directions:

1. Spray 8 cups muffin pan with cooking spray and set aside.
2. Insert wire rack in rack position 6. Select bake, set temperature 350 f, timer for 30 minutes. Press start to preheat the oven.
3. Add all ingredients into the mixing bowl and whisk well.
4. Pour mixture into the prepared muffin pan and bake for 30 minutes.
5. Serve and enjoy.

12. Mouthwatering Shredded BBQ Roast

Total time: 40 min

Prep time: 10 min

Cook time: 30 min

Yield: 8 servings

Ingredients:

- 4 lbs. Pork roast
- 1 tsp. Garlic powder
- Salt and pepper to taste
- 1/2 cup water
- 2 can (11 oz.) Of barbecue sauce, keno unsweetened

Directions:

1. Season the pork with garlic powder, salt and pepper, place in your instant pot.
2. Pour water and lock lid into place; set on the meat/stew, the high-pressure setting for 30 minutes.
3. When ready, use quick release - turn the valve from sealing to venting to release the pressure.
4. Remove pork in a bowl, and with two forks, shred the meat.
5. Pour BBQ sauce and stir to combine well.
6. Serve.

13.Sour and Spicy Spareribs

Total time: 50 min

Prep time: 15 min

Cook time: 35 min

Yield: 10 servings

Ingredients:

- 5 lbs. Spare spareribs
- Salt and pepper to taste
- 2 tbsp. Of tallow
- 1/2 cup coconut amines (from coconut sap)
- 1/2 cup vinegar
- 2 tbsp. Worcestershire sauce, to taste
- 1 tsp. Chili powder

- 1 tsp. Garlic powder
- 1 tsp. Celery seeds

Directions:

1. Break into similar parts the rack of ribs.
2. Season the spareribs on both sides with salt and ground pepper.
3. In your instant pot, add tallow and put the spareribs.
4. Mix all the remaining ingredients in a cup and spill over the spareribs.
5. Click the lid in place and set it to heat for 35 minutes on the manual setting.
6. Click "cancel" as the timer beeps, then flip the natural release gently for 20 minutes.
7. Open the cover and put the ribs on a serving tray.
8. Serve it hot.

14.Tender Pork Shoulder with Hot Peppers

Prep time: 10 minutes

Cook time: 30 minutes

Yield: 8 servings

Ingredients:

- 3 lbs. Pork shoulder boneless
- Salt and ground black pepper to taste
- 3 tbsp. Of olive oil
- 1 large onion, chopped
- 2 cloves garlic minced
- 2 - 3 chili peppers, chopped
- 1 tsp. Ground coriander
- 1 tsp. ground cumin
- 1 ½ cups of bone broth (preferably homemade)

- 1/2 cup water

Directions:

1. Season the salt and the pork meat with pepper.

2. Switch the instant pot on and press the button to sauté. When the term 'heat' appears on the show, add the oil and sauté for around 5 minutes with the onions and garlic.

3. Add the pork and cook on both sides for 1 - 2 minutes; turn off the sauté button.

4. In an instant kettle, add all the remaining ingredients.

5. Click the lid in place and set it on high heat for 30 minutes on the meat/stew level.

6. Click "cancel" as the timer beeps, then flip the natural release button gently for 15 minutes. Serve it warm.

15.Braised Sour Pork Filet

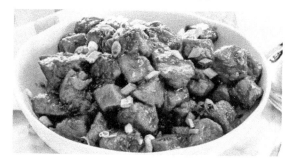

Prep time: 10 minutes

Cook time: 8 hours

Yield: 6 servings

Ingredients:

- 1/2 tsp. Of dry thyme

- 1/2 tsp. Of sage

- Salt and ground black pepper to taste

- 2 tabs of olive oil

- 3 lbs. Of pork fillet
- 1/3 cup of shallots (chopped)
- Three cloves of garlic (minced)
- 3/4 cup of bone broth
- 1/3 cup of apple cider vinegar

Directions:

1. Combine the thyme, sage, salt and black ground pepper in a shallow cup.
2. Rub the pork generously on both edges.
3. In a large frying pan, heat the olive oil and cook the pork for 2 - 3 minutes.
4. Place the pork and add the shallots and garlic in your crockpot.
5. Sprinkle with broth and apple cider vinegar/juice.
6. Cover and simmer for 8 hours on slow heat or 4-5 hours on high heat.
7. Change the salt and pepper, slice and serve with cooking juice and cut the pork from the pan.

16.Pork with Anise and Cumin Stir-Fry

Total time: 35 min

Prep time: 5 min

Cook time: 30 min

Yield: 4 servings

Ingredients:

- 2 tbsp. Lard
- 2 spring onions finely chopped (only green part)
- 2 cloves garlic, finely chopped
- 2 lbs. Pork loin, boneless, cut into cubes
- Sea salt and black ground pepper to taste

- 1 green bell pepper (cut into thin strips)
- 1/2 cup water
- 1/2 tsp. Dill seeds
- 1/2 anise seeds
- 1/2 tsp. Cumin

Directions:

1. Heat the lard n a large frying pot over medium-high heat.
2. Sauté the spring onions and garlic with a pinch of salt for 3 - 4 minutes.
3. Add the pork and simmer for about 5 - 6 minutes.
4. Add all remaining ingredients: and stir well.
5. Cover and let simmer for 15 - 20 minutes
6. Taste and adjust seasoning to taste.
7. Serve!

17. Baked Meatballs with Goat Cheese

Total time: 50 min

Prep time: 15 min

Cook time: 35 min

Yield: 8 servings

Ingredients:

- 1 tbsp. Of tallow
- 2 lbs. Of ground beef
- 1 organic egg
- 1 grated onion
- 1/2 cup of almond milk (unsweetened)
- 1 cup of red wine
- 1/2 bunch of chopped parsley

- 1/2 cup of almond flour
- Salt and ground pepper to taste
- 1/2 tbsp. Of dry oregano
- 4 oz. Of hard goat cheese cut into cubes

Directions:

1. Preheat oven to 400°f.
2. Grease a baking pan with tallow.
3. In a large bowl, combine all ingredients except goat cheese.
4. Knead the mixture until ingredients: are evenly combined.
5. Make small meatballs and place them in a prepared baking dish.
6. Place one cube of cheese on each meatball.
7. Bake for 30 - 35 minutes.
8. Serve hot.

18.Parisian Schnitzel

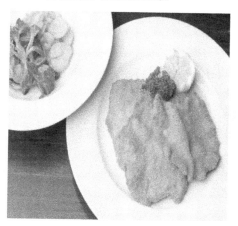

Total time: 25 min

Prep time: 15 min

Cook time: 10 min

Yield: 4 servings

Ingredients:

- Four veal steaks; thin schnitzel
- Salt and ground black pepper
- 2 tbsp. Of butter
- Three eggs from free-range chickens
- 4 tbsp. Of almond flour

Directions:

1. With salt and pepper, season the steaks.
2. Heat butter over medium heat in a large nonstick frying pan.
3. Beat the eggs in a bowl.
4. In a bowl, add the almond flour.

5. Using almond flour to roll each steak, then add and dip in the beaten eggs.

6. Fry each side for around 3 minutes.

7. Serve instantly.

19.Kato Beef Stroganoff

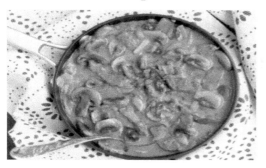

Prep time: 5 minutes

Cook time: 30 minutes

Yield: 6 servings

Ingredients:

- 2 lbs. Of rump or round steak or stewing steak
- 4 tbsp. Of olive oil
- 2 green onions, finely chopped
- 1 grated tomato
- 2 tbsp. Ketchup (without sugar)
- 1 cup of button mushrooms
- 1/2 cup of bone broth
- 1 cup of sour cream
- Salt and black pepper to taste

Directions:

1. Break the beef into strips and sauté it in a large pan for frying.

2. Add the chopped onion and a pinch of salt and roast at a medium temperature for around 20 minutes.

3. Add the ketchup and mushrooms and mix for 3 - 5 minutes.

4. Pour the sour cream and bone broth and simmer for 3 to 4 minutes.

5. Remove and taste from the fire and change the salt and pepper to taste.

6. Serve it warm.

20. Meatloaf with Gruyere

Total time: 55 min

Prep time: 15 min

Cook time: 40 min

Yields: 6 servings

Ingredients:

- 1 1/2 lbs. Ground beef
- 1 cup ground almonds
- 1 large egg from free-range chickens
- 1/2 cup grated gruyere cheese
- 1 tsp. Fresh parsley finely chopped
- 1 scallion finely chopped
- 1/2 tsp. Ground cumin
- 3 eggs boiled
- 2 tbsp. Of fresh grass-fed butter, melted

Directions:

1. Preheat the oven to 350 degrees F.

2. Combine all the ingredients in a large bowl (except for the eggs and butter).

3. Use your hands to combine the mixture properly.

4. Shape the mixture into a roll and put the sliced hard-boiled eggs in the middle.

5. To a 5x9 inch loaf pan greased with melted butter, switch the meatloaf.

6. Put in the oven and cook for 40 minutes, or until the temperature inside is 160 °F.

7. Take it out of the oven and let it sit for 10 minutes.

8. Slicing and cooking.

9.

21.Roasted Filet Mignon in Foil

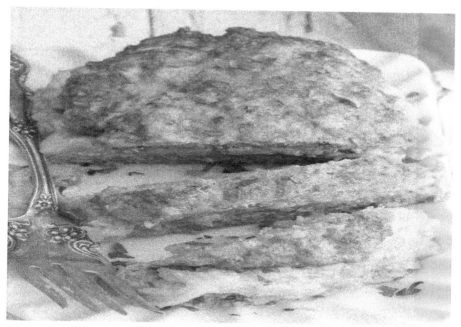

Total time: 60 min

Prep time: 15 min

Cook time: 45 min

Yield: 8 servings

Ingredients:

- 3 lbs. Filet mignon in one piece
- Salt to taste and ground black pepper
- 1 tsp. Of garlic powder
- 1 tsp. Of onion powder
- 1 tsp. Of cumin
- 4 tbsp. Of olive oil

Directions:

1. Preheat the oven to 425°f.

2. Rinse and clean the filet mignon, removing all fats, or ask your butcher to do it for you.

3. Season with salt and pepper, garlic powder, onion powder and cumin.

4. Wrap filet mignon in foil and place in a roasting pan, drizzle with the olive oil.

5. Roast for 15 minutes per pound for medium-rare or to desired doneness.

6. Remove from the oven and allow to rest for 10 -15 minutes before serving.

22.Stewed Beef with Green Beans

Prep time: 10 minutes

Cook time: 50 minutes

Yield: 8 servings

Ingredients:

- 1/2 cup olive oil
- 1 1/2 lbs. Beef cut into cubes
- 2 scallions, finely chopped
- 2 cups water
- 1 lb. Fresh green beans - trimmed and cut diagonally in half
- 1 bay leaf
- 1 grated tomato
- 1/2 cup fresh mint leaves, finely chopped
- 1 tsp. Fresh or dry rosemary
- Salt and freshly ground pepper to taste

Directions:

1. Chop the beef into cubes that are 1 inch thick.

2. In a big pot, heat olive oil over high heat. Sauté the beef and sprinkle it with a pinch of salt and pepper for around 4 - 5 minutes.

3. Add the scallions and mix and sauté until softened for around 3 - 4 more minutes. For 2-3 minutes, pour water and cook.

4. Add the grated tomato and bay leaf. Cook for 5 minutes or so; reduce the heat to medium-low. For about 15 minutes, cover and boil.

5. Add the rosemary, green beans, salt, fresh ground pepper and ample water to cover all the ingredients. Simmer softly, until the green beans are tender, for 15 - 20 minutes.

6. Sprinkle with the rosemary and mint, carefully blend and extract from the sun. Serve it warm.

23.Garlic Herb Butter Roasted Radishes

Total time: 20 min

Prep time: 10 min

Cook time: 10 min

Yield: (4per servings)

Ingredients:

- 1-pound of radishes
- 2 tablespoons of unsalted butter, melted
- 1/2 teaspoon of garlic powder
- ½ teaspoon of dried parsley
- 1/4 teaspoon of dried oregano
- 1/4 teaspoon of ground black pepper

Directions:

1. Separate the roots from the radishes and cut them into parts.

2. Then, in a small bowl, spread butter and seasonings. Swirl the radishes in the herbal butter and place them in the Air Fryer basket.

3. Fix the temperature for 10 minutes to 350° F and adjust the timer.

4. Throw the radishes halfway through the cooking cycle in the Air Fryer basket. Enable it to cool until the edges begin to turn orange.

5. Serve it hot and drink it!

24. Sausage-Stuffed Mushroom Caps

Total time: 20 min

Prep time: 10 min

Cook time: 10 min

Yield: (4per servings)

Ingredients:

- 6 large portobello mushroom caps
- ½-pound of Italian sausage
- 1/4 cup of chopped onion
- 2 tablespoons of blanched finely ground almond flour
- ¼ cup of grated Parmesan cheese
- 1 teaspoon of minced fresh garlic

Directions:

1. To hollow each cap of the mushrooms, use a spoon and save the scraps.

2. Brown the sausage for approximately 10 minutes in a medium saucepan over medium pressure,

3. Or until completely cooked and there is no residual pink. Drain the mushroom, cabbage, almond flour, parmesan, and garlic and then add preserved scrapings. Gently fold the ingredients together and proceed to cook for another minute, then extract them from the flames.

4. Scoop the mixture equally into mushroom caps and put the caps in a bowl of 6 rounds. Place the pan in an Air Fryer basket.

5. Set the temperature to 375° F and set the eight-minute timer.

6. When frying is finished, the tops will be browned and bubbled, and serve gently.

25.Cheesy Cauliflower Tots

Total time: 20 min

Prep time: 10 min

Cook time: 10 min

Yield: (4per servings)

Ingredients:

- 1 large head of cauliflower
- 1 cup of shredded mozzarella cheese
- 1/2 cup of grated Parmesan cheese
- 1large egg
- 1/4 teaspoon of garlic powder
- 1/4 teaspoon of dried parsley
- 1/8 teaspoon of onion powder

Directions:

1. On the stovetop, fill a huge pot with 2 cups of water and place a steamer in the oven. Get the bath to a boil. Break the cauliflower into a flower and put the pot and lid on a steamer box.

2. Let the cauliflower steam for 7 minutes, until tender. Place the steamer basket in your cheesecloth or clean kitchen towel and let it cool. To remove as much excess humidity as possible, push on the sink. The mixture would be too fragile to form into tots if not all of the moisture is extracted. Mash down with a razor into a smooth consistency.

3. Place the cauliflower and add the mozzarella, parmesan, cheese, garlic powder, parsley, and onion powder in a large

mixing cup. Remove before you mix properly. Smooth but easy to mold, the mix should be.

4. Roll the mixture into a tot shape by taking 2 teaspoons of the mixture. Repeat for the remaining mixture. In the Air Fryer, bring the basket in.

5. Fix the temperature for 12 minutes to 320° F and set the timer.

6. Switch the tots halfway through the cooking time. Cauliflower tots, when fully baked, should be golden. Serve it hot.

26.Crispy Brussels sprouts

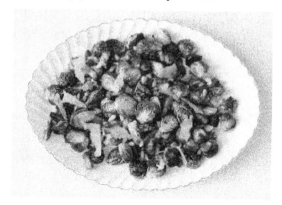

Total time: 20 min

Prep time: 10 min

Cook time: 10 min

Yield: (4per servings)

Ingredients:

- 1-pound of Brussels sprouts
- 1 tablespoon of coconut oil
- 1 tablespoon of unsalted butter, melted

Directions:

1. Every sprout of loose leaves from Brussels is removed and cut in half.

2. Spray it with coconut oil and drop it in the Air Fryer basket.

3. Set the temperature to 400 degrees F and for 10 minutes, change the timer. Depending on how they start browning, you might want to stir gently halfway through the cooking process.

4. When fully baked, they should be tender with darker caramelized spots. Drizzle with the molten butter and cut it out of the bowl of the fryer. Serve without hesitation.

27.Zucchini Parmesan Chips

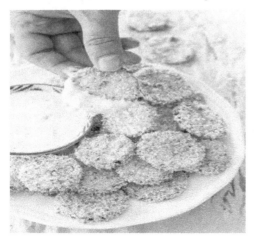

Total time: 20 min

Prep time: 10 min

Cook time: 10 min

Yield: 1 serving

Ingredients:

- 2 medium zucchinis
- 1-ounce of pork rinds
- 1/2 cup of grated Parmesan cheese
- 1 large egg

Directions:

1. 1/4-inch thick slices of a zucchini slice. To extract the excess moisture, place 30 minutes between two layers of paper towels or a clean kitchen towel.

2. In a food processor, put pork rinds and pulse until finely ground. Pour into a medium bowl and blend with parmesan.

3. In a small saucepan, pound the potato.

4. In the egg mixture, dip the zucchini slices and then cover as deeply as possible in the pork rind mixture. Put each slice

46

carefully in a single layer of the Air Fryer bowl, working in batches as needed.

5. Adjust the temperature and set a 10-minute timer to 320° F.

6. Halfway into cooking time, flip chips. Serve hot and enjoy!

28.Roasted Garlic

Total time: 20 min

Prep time: 10 min

Cook time: 10 min

Yield: 1 serving

Ingredients:

- 1 medium head of garlic
- 2 teaspoons of avocado oil

Directions:

1. Strip any excess peel hanging from the garlic still cover the cloves. Shutdown

1/4 of the garlic handle, with clove tips visible.

2. Avocado oil spray. Place the garlic head in a small sheet of aluminum foil, and enclose it completely. Place it in the basket for Air Fryer.

3. Set the temperature to 400° F and change the timer for 20 minutes. If your garlic head is a little smaller, take 15 minutes to check it out.

4. Ail should be golden brown and very fluffy when finished.

5. Cloves should pop out to eat and be scattered or sliced quickly. In the refrigerator, lock in an airtight jar for up to 5 days. You can also freeze individual cloves on a baking sheet, then lock them together until frozen in a freezer-safe storage jar.

29.Kale Chips

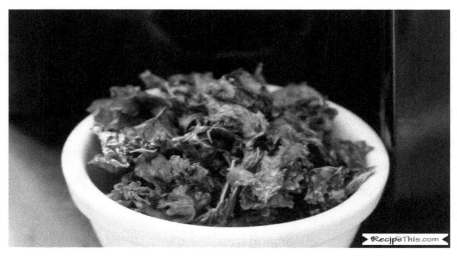

Total time: 20 min

Prep time: 10 min

Cook time: 10 min

Yield: 2 servings

Ingredients:

- 4 cups of steamed kale
- 2 teaspoons of avocado oil
- 1/2 teaspoon of salt

Directions:

1. Sprinkle the kale in a big bowl of avocado oil and sprinkle it with ice. Place it inside the Air Fryer basket.
2. Adjust the temperature and set a 5-minute timer to 400° f.

3. The kale will be crispy until it was done. Serve without hesitation.

30.Buffalo Cauliflower

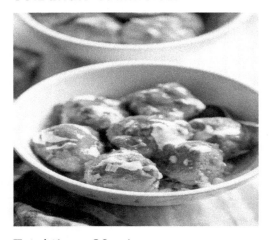

Total time: 20 min

Prep time: 10 min

Cook time: 10 min

Yield: 4 servings

Ingredients:

- 4 cups of cauliflower florets
- 2 tablespoons of salted butter, melted
- 1/2 (1-ounce)dry ranch seasoning packet
- 1/4 cup of buffalo sauce

Directions:

1. Toss the cauliflower with the butter and dry the ranch in a wide bowl. Place the basket in the Air Fryer.

2. Change the temperature and set the timer to 400°F for 5 minutes.

3. Shake the basket during the cooking process two to three times. Remove the coli flower from the fryer basket when tender and toss in the buffalo sauce. Serve it hot.

31. Green Bean Casserole

Total time: 20 min

Prep time: 10 min

Cook time: 10 min

Yield: 4 servings

Ingredients:

- 4 tablespoons of unsalted butter
- 1/4 cup of diced yellow onion
- 1/2 cup of chopped white mushrooms
- 1/2 cup of heavy whipping cream
- 1 ounce of full-Fat: cream cheese
- 1/2 cup of chicken broth
- 1/4 teaspoon of xanthan gum 1-pound fresh green beans, edges trimmed
- ½ ounce of pork rinds, finely ground

Directions:

1. Melt butter over low heat in a medium saucepan. Before they become soft and fragrant, cook the onion and mushrooms for around 3–5 minutes.

2. Add the hard whipped cream, cream cheese, and broth to the saucepan. Before, whisk quickly. Bring it to a boil, then drop it to a simmer. Sprinkle the gum with xanthan gum in the pan and fry.

3. Break the green beans into 2 parts and arrange them in a round 4-cup baking dish. Spillover those with the sauce mixture and stir until fried. With the rinds of the ground pork, fill the dish.

4. Fix the temperature to 320 degrees F and for 15 minutes, set the timer.

5. Top fork-tender when fully fried, golden and green beans. Soft serving.

32.Cilantro Lime Roasted Cauliflower

Total time: 20 min

Prep time: 10 min

Cook time: 10 min

Yield: 4 servings

Ingredients:

- 2 cups of chopped cauliflower florets
- 2 tablespoons of coconut oil, melted
- 2teaspoons of chili powder
- 1/2 teaspoon of garlic powder
- 1 medium lime
- 2 tablespoons of chopped cilantro

Directions:

1. In a big bowl of coconut oil, combine the cauliflower. Using ground chili and garlic to scatter. Put some seasoned cauliflower in the Air Fryer basket.

2. Set the temperature to 350 degrees F and change the seven-minute timer. The cauliflower gets wet on the sides and starts to turn golden. Set it down in a bowl to eat.

3. Break the lime into quarters and spill over it with cauliflower milk. Coriander garnish.

33.Dinner Rolls

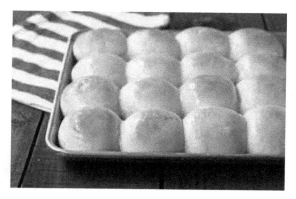

Total time: 20 min

Prep time: 10 min

Cook time: 10 min

Yield: 4 servings

Ingredients:

- 1 cup of shredded mozzarella cheese

- 1 ounce of full-Fat: cream cheese

- 1 cup of blanched finely ground almond flour

- 1/4 cup of ground flaxseed

- ½ teaspoon of baking powder

- 1 large egg

Directions:

1. Place the mozzarella, cream cheese, and almond flour in a large microwave-safe oven. Until flat, blend.

2. Substitute until smooth and thoroughly mixed with flaxseed, baking powder, and egg. Pulse for another 15 seconds if it gets too stiff.

3. Separate the dough into six pieces and roll the dough into balls. Put the Air Fryer balls in the basket.

4. Turn to 320° F and set the 12-minute timer.

5. Enable the rolls to cool completely before eating.

34. Fiery Stuffed Peppers

Preparation time: 20 minutes

Cooking time: 20 minutes

Servings: 4

Ingredients:

- 4 medium green peppers, seeds and stems removed
- 150 g lean minced meat
- 80g grated cheddar cheese, divided
- ½ cup tomato sauce, divided
- ½ tsp. Dried mango powder
- ½ tsp. Chili powder
- ½ tsp. Turmeric powder
- 1 tsp. Worcestershire sauce
- 1 tsp. Coriander powder
- 1 onion, minced
- 1 clove garlic, minced
- 2 tsp., minced coriander leaves
- 1 tsp. Vegetable oil

Directions:

1. Start by setting the oven to 390 degrees f for your air fryer toast.

2. Cook the peppers in salted boiling water for 3 minutes, then move them to a dish.

3. Apply the oil over medium-low heat to a small saucepan and sauté the onion and garlic for 1-2 minutes, then remove from the heat.

4. Combine all the ingredients, except half the cheese and tomato sauce, in a big bowl.

5. With the beef mixture, stuff the peppers and cover with the remaining cheese and tomato sauce.

6. Lightly oil the basket and place the 4 stuffed peppers from your air fryer toast oven.

7. Cook for 15 to 20 minutes or before you want it cooked. Enjoy!

35. Beef and veggies stir fry

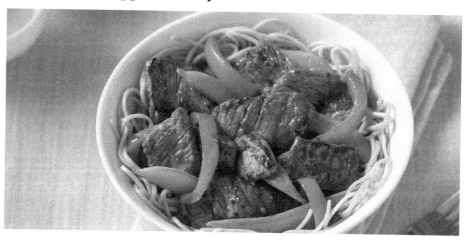

Preparation time: 45 minutes

Cooking time: 15 minutes

Servings: 4

Ingredients:

- 450g beef sirloin, cut into strips

- 1 yellow pepper, sliced

- 1 red pepper, sliced

- 1 green pepper, sliced

- 1 broccoli, cut into florets
- 1 large red onion, sliced
- 1 large white onion, sliced
- 1 tsp. Sesame oil
- For the marinade:
- 2 tsp. Minced garlic
- 1 tbsp. Low sodium soy sauce
- ¼ cup hoisin sauce
- ¼ cup water
- 1 tsp. Sesame oil
- 1 tsp. Ground ginger

Directions:

1. In a wide bowl, begin by whisking all the marinade ingredients. Add in the strips of beef and toss well, so all the bits are covered equally. Using cling wrap to protect it and let it stay for 30 minutes in the fridge.

2. Combine all the vegetables and the sesame oil and place the toast oven in the basket of your air fryer at 200 degrees F. For 5 minutes, cook.

3. Move the vegetables to a bowl and put the meat in your toast oven's air fryer basket.

4. Be sure that the marinade is drained. Increase the temperature and simmer for 5 minutes, to 360 degrees f. Shake the meat and cook for an additional 3 minutes, or until needed.

5. Attach the vegetables and simmer for an extra 2 minutes.

6. Serve on a steamed rice bed. Enjoy!

36.Air Fried Chili Beef with Toasted Cashews

Preparation time: 10 minutes

Cooking time: 25 minutes

Servings: 24

Ingredients:

- ½ tablespoon extra-virgin olive oil or canola oil
- 450g sliced lean beef
- 2 teaspoons red curry paste
- 1 teaspoon liquid stevia, optional
- 2 tablespoons fresh lime juice
- 2 teaspoon fish sauce
- 1 cup green capsicum, diced
- ½ cup water
- 24 toasted cashews
- 1 teaspoon arrowroot starch

Directions:

1. Set the oven to 375 degrees f for your air fryer toast.

2. Mix the beef and olive oil and fry for about 15 minutes until the inside is no longer yellow, rotating twice.

3. Apply the red curry paste and simmer for a few more minutes.

4. Mix the stevia, lime juice, fish sauce, capsicum and water in a big pot; boil for about 10 minutes.

5. To make a paste, mix cooked arrowroot with water; stir the paste into the sauce to thicken it.

6. Attach the fried cashews and remove the pan from the sun. Serve.

37.Beef Stir Fry W/ Red Onions & Peppers

Preparation time: 10 minutes

Cooking time: 10 minutes

Servings: 4

Ingredients:

- 450g grass-fed flank steak, thinly sliced strips
- 1 tablespoon rice wine
- 2 teaspoons balsamic vinegar
- Pinch of sea salt
- Pinch of pepper
- 3 teaspoons extra-virgin olive oil
- 1 large yellow onion, thinly chopped
- 1/2 red bell pepper, thinly sliced
- 1/2 green bell pepper, thinly sliced
- 1 tablespoon toasted sesame seeds
- 1 teaspoon crushed red pepper flakes

Directions:

Place meat in a bowl; stir in rice wine and vinegar, sea salt and pepper. Toss to coat well.

Set your air fryer toast oven to 375 degrees f.

Add the meat and olive and cook for about 3-5 minutes or until the meat is browned.

Heat the remaining oil on a stovetop pan and sauté onions for about 2 minutes or until caramelized; stir in pepper and cook for 2 minutes more.

Add the caramelized onions to the air fryer toast oven and stir in sesame seeds and red pepper flakes and cook for 1-2 minutes. Serve hot!

38.Air Fryer Toast Oven Italian Beef

Preparation time: 10 minutes

Cooking time: 1 hour 30 minutes

Servings: 8

Ingredients:

- 1200g grass-fed chuck roast
- 6 cloves garlic
- 1 tsp. Marjoram
- 1 tsp. Basil
- 1 tsp. Oregano
- 1/2 tsp. Ground ginger
- 1 tsp. Onion powder
- 2 tsp. Garlic powder
- 1 tsp. Salt
- 1/4 cup apple cider vinegar
- 1 cup beef broth

Directions:

1. Cut slits in the roast with a sharp knife and then stuff with garlic cloves. In a bowl, whisk together marjoram, basil, oregano, ground ginger, onion powder, garlic powder, and salt until well blended; rub the seasoning all over the roast and place in a large air fryer toast oven pan.

2. Add vinegar and broth and lock lid; cook at 400 degrees f for 90 minutes. Take the roast out and then shred meat with a fork. Serve along with cooking juices.

39.Healthy Quinoa Bowl with Grilled Steak & Veggies

Preparation time: 10 minutes

Cooking time: 20 minutes

Servings: 4

Ingredients:

- 2 cups quinoa
- 16 ounces steak, cut into bite-size pieces
- 1 cup baby arugula

- 1 cup sweet potato slices

- 1 cup red pepper, chopped

- 1 cup scallions, chopped

- 1/2 cup toasted salted pepitas

- 2 tsp. Fresh cilantro leaves

- 2 cups microgreens

- 2 tbsp. Tomato sauce

- 2 tbsp. Extra-virgin olive oil

- Kosher salt

- Black pepper

- 1 tbsp. Fresh lime juice

Directions:

1. In your instant cooker, cook quinoa as needed.

2. Meanwhile, in your air-fryer toast oven, grill steak to medium rare for around 15 minutes at 350 degrees f. Grill the scallions, red pepper and sweet potatoes until tender, along with the beef.

3. Top with grilled beef, scallions, veggies, pepitas, cilantro, and microgreens. Place cooked quinoa in a bowl.

4. Combine the oil, tomato sauce, salt, and pepper in a small bowl until well blended; drizzle over the steak mixture and serve with lime juice.

27. Pork and Mixed Greens Salad

Preparation time: 10 minutes

Cooking time: 15 minutes

Servings: 4

Ingredients:

- 2 pounds pork tenderloin, slice into 1-inch slices

- 1 teaspoon dried marjoram

- 6 cups mixed salad greens
- 1 (8-ounce) package button mushrooms, sliced
- 1/3 cup low-sodium low-fat vinaigrette dressing

Directions:

1. Combine the olive oil and the pork slices. Toss it to coat it.
2. Sprinkle the marjoram and pepper with them and rub them onto the pork.
3. Grill the pork in batches in an air fryer until the pork on a meat thermometer hits at least 145 °f.
4. Combine the red bell pepper, salad greens, and mushrooms. Gently toss.
5. Add the slices to the salad until cooked.
6. Drizzle and toss softly with the vinaigrette. Immediately serve.

40.Pork Satay

Preparation time: 15 minutes

Cooking time: 14 minutes

Servings: 4

Ingredients:

- 1 (1-pound) pork tenderloin, cut into 1½-inch cubes
- ¼ cup minced onion
- 2 garlic cloves, minced
- 2 tablespoons freshly squeezed lime juice, coconut milk, curry powder
- 2 tablespoons unsalted peanut butter

Directions:

1. Combine the ham, ginger, garlic, jalapeño, coconut milk, lime juice, peanut butter, and curry powder with the mixture. Place it aside at room temperature for 10 minutes.

2. From the marinade, take the pork out. Marinade Reserve.

3. Onto approximately 8 bamboo skewers, string the pork. With the reserved marinade, grill and clean once, before the pork on a meat thermometer hits at least 145 °f. Discard every marinade that exists. Immediately serve.

41.Pork Burgers with Red Cabbage Salad

Preparation time: 20 minutes

Cooking time: 9 minutes

Servings: 4

Ingredients:

- ½ cup greek yogurt

- 2 tablespoons low-sodium mustard, paprika

- 1 tablespoon lemon juice

- ¼ cup red cabbage, carrots

- 1-pound lean ground pork

Directions:

1. Combine 1 tablespoon of mustard, lemon juice, cabbage, and carrots with the yogurt; blend and cool.

2. Combine the bacon, 1 tablespoon of mustard left, and the paprika. Mold into eight little patties.

3. Insert the sliders into the basket of the air fryer. Grill with a meat thermometer until the sliders register 165 ° f as checked.

4. By putting some of the lettuce greens on a bun bottom, arrange the burgers. Cover it with a slice of onion, tacos, and a combination of cabbage. Attach the top of the bun and quickly serve.

42.Crispy Mustard Pork Tenderloin

Preparation time: 10 minutes

Cooking time: 12 to 16 minutes

Servings: 4

Ingredients:

- 3 tablespoons low-sodium grainy mustard
- ¼ teaspoon dry mustard powder
- 1 (1-pound) pork tenderloin
- ¼ cup ground walnuts
- 2 tablespoons cornstarch

Directions:

6. Stir together the mustard, olive oil, and mustard powder. Spread this mixture over the pork.

7. On a plate, mix the bread crumbs, walnuts, and cornstarch. Dip the mustard-coated pork into the crumb mixture to coat.

8. Air-fry the pork until it registers at least 145°f on a meat thermometer. Slice to serve.

43. Apple Pork Tenderloin

Preparation time: 10 minutes

Cooking time: 14 to 19 minutes

Servings: 4

Ingredients:

- 1 (1-pound) pork tenderloin, cut into 4 pieces
- 1 tablespoon apple butter
- 2 granny smith apples or Jonagold apples, sliced
- ½ teaspoon dried marjoram
- 1/3 cup apple juice

Directions:

1. Rub the apple butter and olive oil with each slice of pork.

2. Mix together the bacon, apples, 3 celery, 1 marjoram, 1 cabbage, and apple juice.

3. Place the bowl in the fryer and roast until the pork on a meat thermometer hits at least 145 ° f, and the apples and vegetables are tender. During cooking, stir once. Immediately serve.

44.Espresso-Grilled Pork Tenderloin

Preparation time: 15 minutes

Cooking time: 9 to 11 minutes

Servings: 4

Ingredients:

- 2 teaspoons espresso powder
- 1 teaspoon ground paprika
- ½ teaspoon dried marjoram
- 1 tablespoon honey, lemon juice, brown sugar
- 1 (1-pound) pork tenderloin

Directions:

Combine the brown sugar, marjoram, paprika, and espresso powder.

Stir in the olive oil, lemon juice and honey until well combined.

Spread the honey mixture over the pork and let it rest at room temperature for 10 minutes.

In the air fryer basket, roast the tenderloin until the pork reports at least 145°f on a meat thermometer. To cook, slice the beef.

45.Garlic Lamb Chops with Thyme

Preparation time: 10 minutes

Cooking time: 30 minutes

Servings: 4

Ingredients:

- 4 lamb chops
- 1 garlic clove, peeled

- 1 tbsp. plus
- 2 tsp. olive oil
- ½ tbsp. oregano
- ½ tbsp. thyme
- ½ tsp. salt
- ¼ tsp. black pepper

Directions:

1. Preheat the fryer to 390 f for air. Coat the clove of garlic with 1 tsp. Olive oil and put for 10 minutes in the air fryer. Meanwhile, with the remaining olive oil, combine the herbs and seasonings.

2. Squeeze the hot roasted garlic clove into the herb mixture using a towel or a mitten, and stir to blend. Coat the mixture well with the lamb chops, and put them in the air fryer. For 8 to 12 minutes, cook.

3.

46.Lamb Meatloaf

Preparation time: 15 minutes

Cooking time: 40 minutes

Servings: 4

Ingredients:

- 2 lb. Lamb, ground
- 4 scallions; chopped
- 1 egg
- A drizzle of olive oil
- 2 tbsp. Tomato sauce
- 2 tbsp. Parsley; chopped
- 2 tbsp. Cilantro; chopped
- ¼ tsp. Cinnamon powder
- 1 tsp. Coriander, ground
- 1 tsp. Lemon juice
- ½ tsp. Hot paprika
- 1 tsp. Cumin, ground
- A pinch of salt and black pepper

Directions:

1. Combine the lamb in a bowl with the rest of the ingredients, except for the oil, and mix very well.

2. Grease a loaf pan that suits the oil in the air fryer, add the lamb mix and mold the meatloaf

3. Place the pan in an air fryer and cook for 35 minutes at 380 °f. Slicing and serving

4.

47.Lamb Chops and Mint Sauce

Preparation time: 10 minutes

Cooking time: 29 minutes

Servings: 4

Ingredients:

- 8 lamb chops
- 1 cup mint; chopped
- 1 garlic clove; minced
- 2 tbsp. Olive oil
- Juice of 1 lemon
- A pinch of salt and black pepper

Directions:

1. Combine all the ingredients in a blender, except the lamb, and pulse well.
2. Rub lamb chops with the mint sauce, place them in your air fryer's basket and cook at 400°f for 12 minutes on each side
3. Divide and serve everything between plates.

4.

48.Rosemary Roasted Lamb Cutlets

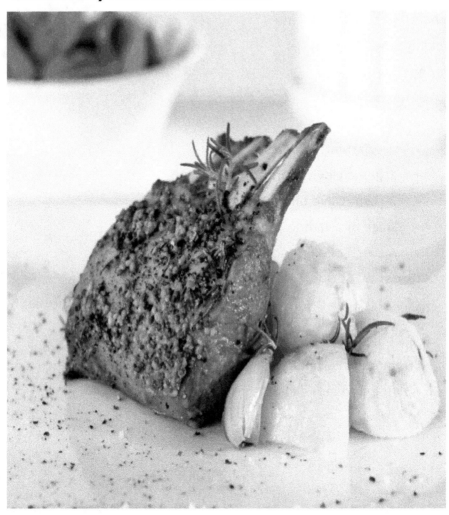

Preparation time: 15 minutes

Cooking time: 35 minutes

Servings: 4

Ingredients:

- 8 lamb cutlets

- 2 garlic cloves; minced
- 2 tbsp. Rosemary; chopped
- 2 tbsp. Olive oil
- A pinch of salt and black pepper
- A pinch of cayenne pepper

Directions:

1. Take a bowl and mix the rest of the ingredients with the lamb: rub well.

2. Place the lamb in the fryer's basket and cook for 30 minutes at 380°f, flipping halfway. Divide between plates and serve the cutlets

49.Seasoned Lamb

Preparation time: 15 minutes

Cooking time: 40 minutes

Servings: 4

Ingredients:

- 1 lb. Lamb leg; boneless and sliced
- ½ cup walnuts; chopped
- 2 garlic cloves; minced
- 1 tbsp. Parsley; chopped
- 1 tbsp. Rosemary; chopped
- 2 tbsp. Olive oil
- ¼ tsp. Red pepper flakes
- ½ tsp. Mustard seeds
- ½ tsp. Italian seasoning
- A pinch of salt and black pepper

Directions:

1. Take a bowl and combine the lamb with all the ingredients: rub well except the walnuts and parsley, place the slices in

69

the basket of your air fryer and cook for 35 minutes at 370 ° F, flipping the meat halfway.

2. Spread the parsley and walnuts on top and serve with a side salad. Split between dishes.

50. Herbed Lamb

Preparation time: 15 minutes

Cooking time: 40 minutes

Servings: 4

Ingredients:

- 8 lamb cutlets
- ¼ cup mustard
- 2 garlic cloves; minced
- 1 tbsp. Oregano; chopped
- 1 tbsp. Mint chopped.
- 1 tbsp. Chives; chopped
- 1 tbsp. Basil; chopped
- A drizzle of olive oil
- A pinch of salt and black pepper

Directions:

1. Take a bowl and mix the rest of the ingredients with the lamb: rub well.

2. Place the cutlets in the basket of your air fryer and cook on each side at 380°f for 15 minutes.

3. Divide and serve with a side salad between dishes.

51. Rack of Lamb

Preparation time: 5 minutes

Cooking time: 10 minutes

Servings: 2 to 4

Ingredients:

- 1 rack of lamb
- 2 tbsp. Of dried rosemary
- 1 tbsp. Of dried thyme
- 2 tsp. Of minced garlic
- Salt
- Pepper
- 4 tbsp. Of olive oil

Directions:

1. Start by combining the herbs, mixing the rosemary, thyme, garlic, salt, pepper, and olive oil in a small bowl and combine well.

2. Rub the mixture all over the lamb, then. Place the lamb rack inside the air fryer. Set the temperature for about 10 minutes, to 360f.

3. After 10 minutes, use the method above to calculate the internal temperature of the lamb rack. It will be 145 f if you want an uncommon one.

4. That will be 160 f if you want a medium. If you'd like to do well, it would be 170 f. Remove the bowls, then serve.

52.Lamb Sirloin Steak

Preparation time: 40 minutes

Cooking time: 15 minutes

Servings: 2 to 4

Ingredients:

- ½ onions
- 4 slices of ginger
- 5 cloves of garlic
- 1 tsp. of garam masala
- 1 tsp. Of ground fennel

- 1 tsp. Of ground cinnamon
- ½ tsp. Of ground cardamom
- 1 tsp. Of cayenne
- 1 tsp. Of salt
- 1 lb. Of boneless lamb sirloin steaks

Directions:

1. Add all the ingredients to a blender bowl, except the lamb chops.
2. Pulse and blend until the onion and all ingredients are finely minced: blend for around 3 to 4 minutes.
3. Place the chops of the lamb into a side dish. To allow the marinade to penetrate better, use a knife to slice the meat and fat.
4. Toss well the mixed spice paste and combine well. Enable the mixture to rest for 30 minutes or in the refrigerator for up to 24 hours.
5. For about 15 minutes, allow your air fryer to 330 f and place the lamb steaks in the air fryer basket in a single layer and cook, flipping halfway through.
6. Ensure that the meat has reached an inner temperature of 150f for medium-well, using a meat thermometer, and serve.

53.Beef Pork Meatballs

Preparation time: 10 minutes

Cooking time: 20 minutes

Servings: 6

Ingredients:

- 1 lb. Ground beef
- 1 lb. Ground pork
- 1/2 cup Italian breadcrumbs

- 1/3 cup milk
- 1/4 cup onion, diced
- 1/2 teaspoon garlic powder
- 1 teaspoon Italian seasoning
- 1 egg
- 1/4 cup parsley chopped
- 1/4 cup shredded parmesan
- Salt and pepper to taste

Directions:

1. In a bowl, carefully mix the beef with all the other meatball ingredients.
2. Create tiny meatballs out of this combination, then put them in the basket of the air fryer.
3. Click the Air Fry Oven control button and switch the knob to pick the bake mode.
4. To set the cooking time to 20 minutes, click the time button and change the dial once again.
5. Now press the temp button to set the temperature at 400 degrees f and rotate the dial.
6. When preheated, put the basket of meatballs in the oven and close the lid.
7. When baked, turn the meatballs halfway through and then start cooking.
8. Serve it hot.

54. Beef Noodle Casserole

Preparation time: 10 minutes

Cooking time: 35 minutes

Servings: 6

Ingredients:

- 2 tablespoons olive oil
- 1 medium onion, chopped
- ½ lb. Ground beef
- 4 fresh mushrooms, sliced
- 1 cup pasta noodles, cooked
- 2 cups marinara sauce
- 1 teaspoon butter
- 4 teaspoons flour
- 1 cup milk
- 1 egg, beaten
- 1 cup cheddar cheese, grated

Directions:

9. Put a wok on moderate heat and add oil to heat.

10. Toss in onion and sauté until soft.

11. Stir in mushrooms and beef, then cook until meat is brown.

12. Add marinara sauce and cook it to a simmer.

13. Stir in pasta then spread this mixture in a casserole dish.

14. Prepare the sauce by melting butter in a saucepan over moderate heat.

15. Stir in flour and whisk well, pour in the milk.

16. Mix well and whisk ¼ cup sauce with egg, then return it to the saucepan.

17. Stir, cook for 1 minute, then pour this sauce over the beef.

18. Drizzle cheese over the beef casserole.

19. Press the "power button" of the air fry oven and turn the dial to select the "bake" mode.

20. Press the time button and again turn the dial to set the cooking time to 30 minutes.

21. Now push the temp button and rotate the dial to set the temperature at 350 degrees f.

22. Once preheated, place the casserole dish in the oven and close its lid.

23. Serve warm.

55.Saucy Beef Bake

Preparation time: 10 minutes

Cooking time: 36 minutes

Servings: 6

Ingredients:

- 2 tablespoons olive oil
- 1 large onion, diced
- 2 lbs. Ground beef
- 2 teaspoons salt
- 6 cloves garlic, chopped
- 1/2 cup red wine
- 6 cloves garlic, chopped
- 3 teaspoons ground cinnamon
- 2 teaspoons ground cumin
- 2 teaspoons dried oregano
- 1 teaspoon black pepper
- 1 can 28 oz. Crushed tomatoes
- 1 tablespoon tomato paste

Directions:

1. In a bowl, carefully mix the beef with all the other meatball ingredients.

2. Create tiny meatballs out of this combination, then put them in the basket of the air fryer.

3. Click the Air Fry Oven control button and switch the knob to pick the bake mode.

4. To set the cooking time to 20 minutes, click the time button and change the dial once again.

5. Now press the temp button to set the temperature at 400 degrees f and rotate the dial.

6. When preheated, put the basket of meatballs in the oven and close the lid.

7. When baked, turn the meatballs halfway through and then start cooking.

8. Serve it hot.

56.Beets and Arugula Salad

Total time: 20 min

Prep time: 10 min

Cook time: 10 min

Yield: 4 servings

Ingredients:

- 1 and ½ pounds of beets, peeled and quartered
- A drizzle of olive oil
- 2 teaspoons of orange zest, grated
- 2 tablespoons of cider vinegar
- ½ cup of orange juice
- 2 tablespoons of brown sugar
- 2 scallions, chopped
- 2 teaspoons of mustard
- 2 cups of arugula

Directions:

1. Rub the beets with the orange juice and oil, put them in your Air Fryer, and cook at 350 °F for 10 minutes.

2. Move the beet quarters to a bowl, add the scallions, arugula zest, and orange and blend.

3. In a separate dish, blend the sugar with the mustard and vinegar, blend properly, add the lettuce, whisk and eat.

57.Beet Tomato and Goat Cheese Mix

Total time: 45 min

Prep time: 20 min

Cook time: 25 min

Yield: 8 servings

Ingredients:

- 8 small beets, trimmed, peeled, and halved
- 1 red onion, sliced
- 4 ounces of goat cheese, crumbled
- 1 tablespoon of balsamic vinegar
- Salt and black pepper to the taste
- 2 tablespoons of sugar
- 1-pint mixed cherry tomatoes halved
- 2 ounces of pecans
- 2 tablespoons of olive oil

Directions:

1. Connect the beets to the Air Fryer, season with salt and pepper, cook for 14 minutes at 350 °F and move to a salad bowl.

2. Attach the carrot, pecans, and cherry tomatoes, and toss.

3. Mix the vinegar with the sugar and oil in another dish, stir well until the sugar dissolves, and add to the salad.

4. Add goat cheese as well, toss, and eat.

58.Broccoli Salad

Total time: 20 min

Prep time: 10 min

Cook time: 10 min

Yield: 8 servings

Ingredients:

- 1 broccoli head, florets separated
- 1 tablespoon of peanut oil
- 6 garlic cloves, minced
- 1 tablespoon of Chinese rice wine vinegar
- Salt and black pepper to the taste

Directions:

1. In a cup, mix broccoli with salt, pepper and half the oil, shake, switch to your Air Fryer, and cook at 350 °F for 8 minutes, shaking halfway through the fryer.
2. Transfer the broccoli and the leftover peanut oil, garlic and rice vinegar into a salad bowl, blend well and eat very nicely.

59.Brussels Sprouts and Tomatoes Mix

Total time: 15 min

Prep time: 5 min

Cook time: 10 min

Yield: 4 servings

Ingredients:

- 1-pound of Brussels sprouts, trimmed
- Salt and black pepper to the taste
- 6 cherry tomatoes, halved
- ¼ cup of green onions, chopped
- 1 tablespoon of olive oil

Directions:

1. Season Brussels with salt and pepper sprouts, put in your fryer and cook at 350 degrees F for 10 minutes.

2. Add salt, pepper, cherry tomatoes, olive oil, and green onions, blend well and eat. Put them in a cup.

60. Brussels Sprouts and Butter Sauce

Total time: 15 min

Prep time: 5 min

Cook time: 10 min

Yield: 4 servings

Ingredients:

- 1-pound of Brussels sprouts, trimmed
- Salt and black pepper to the taste
- ½ cup of bacon, cooked and chopped
- 1 tablespoon of mustard
- 1 tablespoon of butter
- 2 tablespoons dill, finely chopped

Directions:

1. In the Air Fryer, put the Brussels sprouts and cook them at 350 °F for 10 minutes.
2. Heat a skillet with the butter over medium-high heat, add the bacon, mustard, and dill and whisk well.
3. In Brussels, split the sprouts between bowls, drizzle the butter sauce all over, and eat.

61. Cheesy Brussels sprouts

Total time: 18 min

Prep time: 5 min

Cook time: 10 min

Yield: 4 servings

Ingredients:

- 1-pound of Brussels sprouts washed
- Juice of 1 lemon

- Salt and black pepper to the taste
- 2 tablespoons of butter
- 3 tablespoons of parmesan, grated

Directions:

1. Put the sprouts in the Brussels Air Fryer, cook them at 350 degrees F for 8 minutes, and position them on a tray.
2. Heat the butter in a skillet over medium heat, add the lemon juice, salt and pepper, stir well and add the Brussels sprouts.
3. Before the parmesan melts, add the parmesan, toss and serve.

62.Spicy Cabbage

Total time: 18 min

Prep time: 5 min

Cook time: 10 min

Yield: 4 servings

Ingredients:

- 1 cabbage, cut into 8 wedges
- 1 tablespoon of sesame seed oil
- 1 carrot, grated
- ¼ cup of apple cider vinegar
- ¼ cups of apple juice
- ½ teaspoon of cayenne pepper
- 1 teaspoon of red pepper flakes, crushed

Directions:

1. Combine cabbage with oil, carrot, vinegar, apple juice, cayenne, and pepper flakes, shake, put in preheated Air Fryer, and cook for 8 minutes at 350° F in a pan that suits your Air Fryer.

2. Divide and serve cabbage mixture on bowls.

63.Sweet Baby Carrots Dish

Total time: 20 min

Prep time: 5 min

Cook time: 15 min

Yield: 4 servings

Ingredients:

- 2 cups of baby carrots
- A pinch of salt and black pepper
- 1 tablespoon of brown sugar
- ½ tablespoon of butter, melted

Directions:

1. In a dish that fits your Air Fryer blend, add baby carrots with butter, salt, pepper and sugar, place in your Air Fryer, and cook at 350 °F for 10 minutes.
2. Divide and feed between bowls.

64. Collard Greens Mix

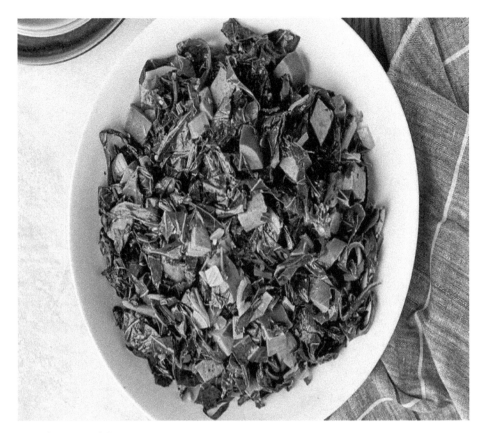

Total time: 20 min

Prep time: 5 min

Cook time: 15 min

Yield: 4 servings

Ingredients:

- 1 bunch of collard greens, trimmed
- 2 tablespoons of olive oil
- 2 tablespoons of tomato puree
- 1 yellow onion, chopped
- 3 garlic cloves, minced
- Salt and black pepper to the taste

- 1 tablespoon of balsamic vinegar
- 1 teaspoon of sugar

Directions:

1. In a bowl that matches your Air Fryer, mix the oil, garlic, vinegar, onion, and tomato puree and whisk.
2. Add the collard greens, salt, pepper and shake with the butter, stir in the Air Fryer and roast at 320 degrees F for 10 minutes.
3. Divide the collard greens into bowls and serve

65.Collard Greens and Turkey Wings

Total time: 30 min

Prep time: 10 min

Cook time: 25 min

Yield: 2 servings

Ingredients:

- 1 sweet onion, chopped
- 2 smoked turkey wings
- 2 tablespoons of olive oil
- 3 garlic cloves, minced
- 2 and ½ pounds of collard greens, chopped
- Salt and black pepper to the taste
- 2 tablespoons of apple cider vinegar
- 1 tablespoon of brown sugar
- ½ teaspoon of crushed red pepper

Directions:

1. Heat up a medium-hot saucepan that suits the grease of your Air Fryer, add the onions, stir and cook for 2 minutes.
2. Connect the garlic, the onions, the mustard, the salt, the pepper, the crushed red pepper, the cinnamon and the

smoked turkey, add the preheated Air Fryer and cook at 350 degrees F for 15 minutes.

66.Herbed Eggplant and Zucchini Mix

Total time: 18 min

Prep time: 5 min

Cook time: 10 min

Yield: 4 servings

Ingredients:

- 1 eggplant, roughly cubed
- 3 zucchinis, roughly cubed
- 2 tablespoons of lemon juice
- Salt and black pepper to the taste
- 1 teaspoon of thyme, dried
- 1 teaspoon of oregano, dried
- 3 tablespoons of olive oil

Directions:

1. Place the eggplant in the bowl of the Air Fryer, add the zucchini, lemon juice, salt, pepper, thyme, oregano and olive oil, blend and place in the Air Fryer and cook for 8 minutes at 360 degrees F.
2. Divide into bowls and instantly serve.

67.Flavored Fennel

Total time: 18 min

Prep time: 5 min

Cook time: 10 min

Yield: 4 servings

Ingredients:

- 2 fennel bulbs, cut into quarters
- 3 tablespoons of olive oil

- Salt and black pepper to the taste
- 1 garlic clove, minced
- 1 red chili pepper, chopped
- ¾ cup of veggie stock
- Juice from ½ lemon
- ¼ cup of white wine
- ¼ cup of parmesan, grated

Directions:

1. Heat a medium-hot saucepan that fits the oil with your Air Fryer, add the garlic and chili pepper, stir and cook for 2 minutes.
2. Add the fennel, salt, pepper, stock, vinegar, lemon juice and parmesan, cover with a swirl, throw in the Air Fryer and cook at 350 °F for 6 minutes.
3. Divide them into plates.

68.Okra and Corn Salad

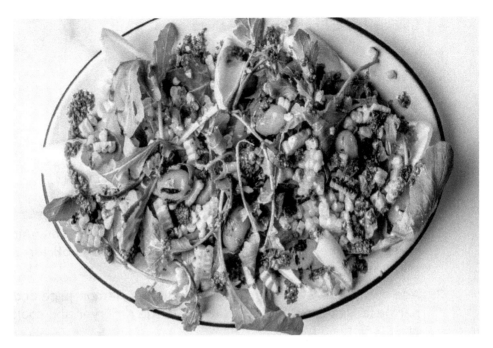

Total time: 20 min

Prep time: 5 min

Cook time: 15 min

Yield: 4 servings

Ingredients:

- 3 green bell peppers, chopped
- 2 tablespoons of olive oil
- 1 teaspoon of sugar
- 1-pound of okra, trimmed
- 6 scallions, chopped
- Salt and black pepper to the taste
- 28 ounces of canned tomatoes, chopped
- 1 cup of corn

Directions:

1. Heat a pan over medium-high heat that suits the oil with your Air Fryer, add bell peppers and scallions, blend and cook for 5 minutes.

2. Connect the okra, salt, pepper, sugar, tomatoes, and maize, stir, put in the Air Fryer and cook at 360 degrees F for 7 minutes.

3. Break the mixture of okra into plates and serve until wet.

69.Air Fried Leeks

Total time: 18 min

Prep time: 5 min

Cook time: 10 min

Yield: 4 servings

Ingredients:

- 4 leeks, washed, ends cut off and halved
- Salt and black pepper to the taste
- 1 tablespoon of butter, melted
- 1 tablespoon of lemon juice

Directions:

1. Rub the leeks with the melted butter, season with salt and pepper, add to the Air Fryer and cook at 350 degrees F for 7 minutes.

2. Set the lemon juice on a pan, drizzle it all over and eat.

70.Crispy Potatoes and Parsley

Total time: 20 min

Prep time: 5 min

Cook time: 15 min

Yield: 4 servings

Ingredients:

- 1-pound of gold potatoes, cut into wedges

- Salt and black pepper to the taste
- 2 tablespoons of olive
- Juice from ½ lemon
- ¼ cup of parsley leaves, chopped

Directions:

1. Rub the potatoes with salt, pepper, lemon juice and olive oil, add them to the Air Fryer and cook at 350 degrees F for 10 minutes.
2. Sprinkle on top of the parsley, break into bowls and eat.

71.Indian Turnips Salad

Total time: 22 min

Prep time: 7 min

Cook time: 15 min

Yield: 4 servings

Ingredients:

- 20 ounces of turnips, peeled and chopped
- 1 teaspoon of garlic, minced
- 1 teaspoon of ginger, grated
- 2 yellow onions, chopped
- 2 tomatoes, chopped
- 1 teaspoon of cumin, ground
- 1 teaspoon of coriander, ground
- 2 green chilies, chopped
- ½ teaspoon of turmeric powder
- 2 tablespoons of butter
- Salt and black pepper to the taste
- A handful of coriander leaves, chopped

Directions:

1. In a saucepan that fits your Air Fryer, heats the butter, melt it, add the green chilies, garlic, and ginger, stir and cook for 1 minute.

2. Add the onions, salt, pepper, tomatoes, turmeric, cumin, cilantro and turnips, stir, put in the Air Fryer and cook at 350 degrees F. for 10 minutes.

3. Break into cups, sprinkle with fresh coriander on top and serve.

72.Simple Stuffed Tomatoes

Total time: 25 min

Prep time: 10 min

Cook time: 15 min

Yield: 6 servings

Ingredients:

- 4 tomatoes, tops cut off and pulp scooped and chopped
- Salt and black pepper to the taste
- 1 yellow onion, chopped
- 1 tablespoon of butter
- 2 tablespoons of celery, chopped
- ½ cup of mushrooms, chopped
- 1 tablespoon of bread crumbs
- 1 cup of cottage cheese
- ¼ teaspoon of caraway seeds
- 1 tablespoon of parsley, chopped

Directions:

1. Heat a saucepan with the butter over medium heat, melt, add the onion and celery, stir and simmer for 3 minutes.

2. Link the mushrooms and tomato pulp and then stir and boil for 1 minute.

3. Add salt, pepper, crumbled bread, cheese, parsley, caraway seeds, stir, cook for another 4 minutes, and heat up.

4. With this blend, stuff the tomatoes, place them in the Air Fryer, and cook at 350 °F for 8 minutes.

5. Divide the stewed tomatoes into bowls and serve.

73.Indian Potatoes

Total time: 22 min

Prep time: 7 min

Cook time: 15 min

Yield: 4 servings

Ingredients:

- 1 tablespoon of coriander seeds
- 1 tablespoon of cumin seeds
- Salt and black pepper to the taste
- ½ teaspoon of turmeric powder
- ½ teaspoon of red chili powder
- 1 teaspoon of pomegranate powder
- 1 tablespoon of pickled mango, chopped
- 2 teaspoons of fenugreek, dried
- 5 potatoes, boiled, peeled, and cubed
- 2 tablespoons of olive oil

Directions:

1. Over medium pressure, heat a saucepan that suits the oil of your Air Fryer, add the coriander and cumin seeds, stir and simmer for 2 minutes.

2. Add cinnamon, pepper, turmeric, chili powder, mango, fenugreek, pomegranate powder and potatoes, blend, add Air Fryer and simmer at 360 °F for 10 minutes.

3. Divide and serve sweetly between bowls.

74.Broccoli and Tomatoes Air Fried Stew

Total time: 30 min

Prep time: 10 min

Cook time: 25 min

Yield: 2 servings

Ingredients:

- 1 broccoli head, florets separated
- 2 teaspoons of coriander seeds
- 1 tablespoon of olive oil
- 1 yellow onion, chopped
- Salt and black pepper to the taste
- A pinch of red pepper, crushed
- 1 small ginger piece, chopped
- 1 garlic clove, minced
- 28 ounces of canned tomatoes, pureed

Directions:

1. Heat a medium-hot pan that matches the oil with your Air Fryer, add the onions, salt, pepper, and red pepper, combine and cook for seven minutes.

2. Add the ginger, garlic, cilantro, tomatoes and broccoli, stir, add to the Air Fryer and cook at 360 degrees F for 12 minutes.

3. Break and serve in pots.

75.Collard Greens and Bacon

Total time: 22 min

Prep time: 7 min

Cook time: 15 min

Yield: 4 servings

Ingredients:

- 1-pound collard greens
- 3 bacon strips, chopped
- ¼ cup cherry tomatoes halved
- 1 tablespoon of apple cider vinegar
- 2 tablespoons of chicken stock
- Salt and black pepper to the taste

Directions:

1. Heat a medium-pressure saucepan, add the bacon, stir and cook for 1-2 minutes.

2. Add the tomatoes, collard greens, vinegar, stock, salt and pepper, blend, add to the Air Fryer and cook at 320 degrees F for 10 minutes.

3. Divide and feed between bowls.

76.Sesame Mustard Greens

Total time: 22 min

Prep time: 7 min

Cook time: 15 min

Yield: 4 servings

Ingredients:

- 2 garlic cloves, minced
- 1-pound of mustard greens, torn
- 1 tablespoon of olive oil
- ½ cup yellow onion, sliced
- Salt and black pepper to the taste
- 3 tablespoons of veggie stock
- ¼ teaspoon of dark sesame oil

Directions:

1. Heat a medium-hot saucepan that suits the grease of your Air Fryer, add the onions, blend and brown for 5 minutes.

2. Add the garlic, stock, onions, salt, and pepper, stir, add to the Air Fryer, and cook at 350 degrees F for 6 minutes.
3. Tie the sesame oil together, swirl to coat, break and serve in cups.

77.Radish Hash

Total time: 18 min

Prep time: 5 min

Cook time: 10 min

Yield: 4 servings

Ingredients:

- ½ teaspoon of onion powder
- 1-pound radishes, sliced
- ½ teaspoon of garlic powder
- Salt and black pepper to the taste
- 4 eggs
- 1/3 cup of parmesan, grated

Directions:

1. In a bowl of salt, pepper, onion and garlic powder, eggs, and parmesan cheese, combine the radishes, then whisk well.
2. Shift the radishes into a fridge-friendly saucepan and simmer at 350° F for 7 minutes.
3. Divide the hash into bowls and serve.

78.Cod Pie with Palmit

Preparation Time: 15 Minutes

Cooking Time: 30 Minutes

Servings: 4-6

Ingredients:

- 2 ¼ lb cod
- 4 ½ lb of natural heart previously grated and cooked

- 12 eggs
- 1 ½ cup olive oil
- 7 oz. of olives
- Tomato Chopped garlic, paprika and sliced onion
- Green seasoning

Directions:

1. In a frying pan, cook the cod and, after cooking, destroy it.

2. Drain the heart of the palm well on the reservation.

3. Along with tomatoes, garlic, paprika, ginger, green seasoning and half of the pitted olives, sauté the cod and palm hearts in olive oil for 20 minutes.

4. Pour 6 eggs into the sample and stir for 5 minutes.

5. Grease the olive oil trays and place the mixture into them.

6. Beat the rest of the eggs and spill over the top evenly.

7. Add tomatoes and olives to garnish.

8. Bake for 40 minutes in the air-fryer at 3800F.

79.Simple and Yummy Cod
Preparation Time: 10 Minutes

Cooking Time: 15 Minutes

Servings: 4-6

Ingredients:

- 2 ¼ lb of desalted cod
- 1 ½ lb of boiled and squeezed potatoes
- 1 can of sour cream
- 2 large onions, sliced
- 1 pot of pitted olive
- ½ cup of olive oil
- Butter for greasing

Directions:

1. In the oil, marinate the onions until they wilt.

2. Give the cod a further 5 minutes to sauté.

3. Add the sour cream and potato and stir for another 5 minutes.

4. Turn the heat off and add some more oil.

5. Place the cod in a refractory greased butter and pass the margarine over it again to render it golden.

6. Bake at 4000F for about 20 minutes or until golden brown in an air fryer.

7. It's fast and delicious to serve with rice.

80.Roasted Tilapia Fillet

Preparation Time: 10 Minutes

Cooking Time: 15 Minutes

Servings: 4-6

Ingredients:

- 2 ¼ lb tilapia fillet
- ½ lemon juice
- 4 sliced tomatoes
- 4 sliced onions
- ½ cup chopped black olives
- 1 pound of boiled potatoes
- 1 tbsp. butter ½ cup sour cream tea
- ½ lb grated mozzarella Olive oil Salt

Directions:

1. With lemon and salt, season the fillets.

2. Place a sheet of onions and tomatoes on an ovenproof tray. On top of the layers, position the fillets.

3. Marinade with another layer of tomato and onion, then the olives and drizzle with the olive oil.

4. Bake in an air-fryer for 15 minutes at 3600F.

5. Squeeze the potatoes in another bowl.

6. Melt the butter in a saucepan. Put the cream with both the potatoes.

7. Place this puree on top of the fillets, then place the mozzarella on top of them.

8. Bake for another 5 minutes in an air fryer at 3600F and serve.

81. Cod 7-Mares
Preparation Time: 10 Minutes

Cooking Time: 15 Minutes

Servings: 4-6

Ingredients:

- 1 lb cod in French fries
- 4 large potatoes, peeled and diced
- 1 can of cream without serum
- 1 cup of coffee with coconut milk
- 3 ½ oz. of mozzarella cheese in strips
- 3 ½ oz. cheese in pieces
- 100 g3 ½ oz. grated Parmesan cheese
- Aromatic herbs and salt to taste.
- 1 tbsp. of curry
- Salt to taste

Directions:

1. Cook and set aside the peeled and diced potatoes.

2. Remove the salt from the cod (leave it overnight in the water and at least change the water

3 times to have the salt erased). 3. Place the potatoes in a glass jar and cook in the microwave for 5 minutes. Set aside.

4. The cream, coconut milk, curry, mozzarella cheese, and herbs are mixed in a bowl. Mounting Up

5. Top a layer of boiled potatoes on a pan, put the cod fries on top, and pour the sauce on top.

6. Season to taste with salt.

7. Sprinkle with Parmesan cheese and cook in an air fryer at 3600F for 7 minutes.

8. Toss the chives over the top when done, and immediately serve.

82.Roasted Hake with Coconut Milk

Preparation Time: 10 Minutes

Cooking Time: 30 Minutes

Servings: 2

Ingredients:

- 2 ¼ lb hake fillet
- ½ lb sliced mozzarella
- 1 can of sour cream
- 1 bottle of coconut milk
- 1 onion
- 1 tomato
- Salt and black pepper to taste.
- Lemon juice

Directions:

1. With salt, pepper and lemon, season the fillets.

2. Let them stand for ten minutes.

3. Arrange the fillets and put each one in the center of the mozzarella slices and roll it up like a fillet.

4. The fillets were rolled up after all.

5. Just get a tray.

6. Place on top of the tomato and onion slices (sliced).

7. Attach the sour cream and coconut milk mixture to the top.

8. Bake for 20 minutes inside an air-fryer at 4000, coated with aluminum foil.

9. Then, to finish baking, remove it.

83.Air fryer Catfish
Preparation Time: 15 Minutes

Cooking Time: 1 Hour

Servings: 2-4

Ingredients:
- 3 pounds sliced dogfish
- 1 pound boiled and sliced potatoes
- 1 package of onion cream
- 3 tomatoes cut into slices
- 3 bell peppers cut into slices
- 3 onions cut into slices
- Olive oil
- 2 garlic cloves, crushed
- Salt to taste
- 1 lemon juice

Directions:

1. With garlic, salt and ginger, season the fish slices and set them aside.

2. Place the potatoes on a baking sheet to get the slices and drizzle with plenty of oil, forming a kind of bed.

3. On the potatoes, spread half of the onion cream.

4. Lay on top of the slices.

5. Place on top of the tomato, bell pepper and onion, spread well and cover the slices. Drizzle with olive oil again, and then pour on top of the rest of the onion cream.

6. Heat the air fryer at 3600F for about 15 minutes and then bake for 1 hour.

84.Squid to the Milanese
Preparation Time: 5 Minutes

Cooking Time: 15 Minutes

Servings: 4-6

Ingredients:

- 2 ¼ lb clean squid
- Salt, pepper and oregano to taste.
- 3 beaten eggs
- 1 cup of wheat flour
- 1 cup breadcrumbs
- 1 cup chopped green chives

Directions:

1. Season the squid with salt, pepper and oregano, after washing and cutting into rings.

2. Put the squid over the beaten eggs, then mix the breadcrumbs with the wheat flour.

3. Fry for 10 minutes in the air-fryer at 4000F. 4. Green onions are sprinkled.

85.Portugal Codfish with Cream
Preparation Time: 10 Minutes

Cooking Time: 15 Minutes

Servings: 2-4

Ingredients:

- 2 ¼ lbs of cod
- 1 chopped onion
- 2 cloves of garlic
- 4 medium potatoes

- 1 leek stalk (Portugal leek)
- 2 cups of cream
- 1 egg Parmesan
- Coriander (optional)
- Olive oil
- Black olives

Directions:

1. Soak the cod in water for approximately 24 hours until the salt is to your taste.

2. Put the oil and brown the garlic, the onion and the leek in a frying pan, then place the cod and let it brown.

3. Take the diced potatoes and cook them separately.

4. Then, with the golden cod, bring the potatoes together. Then put the cilantro along with the cream or sour cream to your liking. Integrate everything.

5. Spread a little Parmesan on top, beat 1 whole egg and sprinkle the cod and marinade with black olives.

6. Place it at 3600F for 30 minutes in an air fryer or until it turns into a crispy cone.

7. Serve with a lovely salad of lettuce, nothing more.

86.Roasted Salmon with Provencal

Preparation Time: 10 Minutes

Cooking Time: 20 Minutes

Servings: 2

Ingredients:

- 4 slices of fresh salmon basil thyme
- Rosemary oregano salt and pepper olive oil
- 4 tablespoons of butter
- ½ lemon juice

Directions:

1. On a hot plate, place the salmon slices and sprinkle with the 4 herbs.

2. Then add salt, pepper and a couple of drops of olive oil to taste.

3. Bake for 15 minutes at 4000F in an air fryer (check every 5 minutes).

4. Serve with potatoes, herbal butter and a new salad.

5. Until it's creamy, whip the butter.

6. Add the same lemon juice and the herbs described previously.

87.Breaded Fish with Tartar Sauce
Preparation Time: 15 Minutes

Cooking Time: 20 Minutes

Servings: 2-4

Ingredients:

- 1 lb of hake fillet
- 4 garlic cloves, crushed
- Juice of 2 lemons
- Salt and black pepper
- Beaten eggs
- Wheat flour
- Vegetable oil for frying

Sauce:

- 3 oz. green olives
- 3 tbsp. chopped onion
- 1 garlic clove, crushed
- Parsley and chives
- 5 tbsp. soy sauce
- ½ can of cream

- 3 tbsp. of dijon mustard
- 1 tbsp. of tomato sauce
- 4 tbsp. mayonnaise

Tartar sauce:
- ½ lb chopped pickles

Directions:

1. Season the fillets with salt, pepper, garlic, and lemon juice, let them taste for at least 30 minutes.

2. Pass the wheat, egg and wheat again.

3. Fry them in the air fryer at 4000F for 25 minutes.

4. Mix all the ingredients in a bowl. 5. Serve with the fillets.

88.Milanese Fish Fillet

Preparation Time: 10 Minutes

Cooking Time: 30 Minutes

Servings: 2-3

Ingredients:

- 1 lb of fish fillet of your choice
- Salt
- 2 garlic cloves, crushed
- 3 eggs Wheat flour
- Oil for frying

Directions:

1. Wash and season the fish fillets with garlic and salt.

2. If you want, you can add the juice of a lemon.

3. Beat the egg whites until stiff and add the egg yolks.

4. Pass the fish fillets, one at a time, in the wheat flour and then pass them over the beaten eggs in the snow.

5. Fry in the air fryer at 4000F for 25 minutes or until they are golden brown.

89.Sole with White Wine

Preparation Time: 10 Minutes

Cooking Time: 35 Minutes

Servings: 4-6

Ingredients:

- 3 lbs of sole fillets
- 5 ¼ oz. of butter
- 1 glass of white wine
- Wheat flour
- Salt black pepper thyme

Directions:

1. Season the fillet with both the wheat flour and pass it on.

2. For 20 minutes or until brown, put in an air fryer at 4000F. In a preheated clay pan, reserve this fish.

3. In the butter, toast a tablespoon of flour.

4. Add the wine to taste, with salt, pepper and thyme. Let everything cook for another three minutes, stirring constantly. Pour the sole over and eat.

90.Golden Fish with Shrimps

Preparation Time: 10 Minutes

Cooking Time: 30 Minutes

Servings: 2-3

Ingredients:

- 1 large golden fish
- 1 lb of shrimp onion
- tomato
- Pepper

- lemon
- olive oil
- Butter
- green smell parsley

Directions:

1. Clean the complete golden and season with lemon, black pepper to taste and salt, the same with the prawns.

2. Leave for 1 hour after seasoning.

3. Place the fish on this plate, add the shrimp to the fish's belly, and tie it with a line. Line a plate with aluminum foil and grease with butter.

4. On top of the gold, put the onion rings, tomatoes and peppers and the green odor with the parsley and use it with plenty of oil.

5. Cover the tray with aluminum foil and bake for 35 minutes at 4000F in the air fryer.

6. With white rice, serve.

91.Stroganoff Cod

Preparation Time: 5 Minutes

Cooking Time: 35 Minutes

Servings: 4-6

Ingredients:

- 1 lb of cod
- 3 tbsp. olive oil
- 2 garlic cloves, minced
- 2 ¼ lb of chopped onion
- 4 ½ lb of skinless tomatoes
- Salt to taste
- ½ cup of brandy
- Oregano, rosemary and black pepper to taste.

- 1 package of chopped green aroma
- 1 cup grated cheese
- 2 ¼ lb of fresh mushrooms cut into chips
- 1 can of sour cream
- 1 large golden fish
- 1 lb of shrimp onion tomato
- Pepper lemon olive oil
- Butter green smell parsley

Directions:

1. Soak the cod in water the day before, boil and crumble all the meat. Reserve. Reserve.

2. In olive oil, saute the onion and garlic. Add the tomatoes that have been chopped and boil until separated. Remove. Remove!

3. Season with salt, oregano, rosemary and black pepper. Blend with the cod and apply the brandy. Add the mushrooms and the green odor.

4. Put it in an air-fryer for 10 minutes at 3200. Taking the fryer out of the air; add the grated cheese and sour cream.

5. Mix well with white rice and serve.

92.Cod Balls

Preparation Time: 10 Minutes

Cooking Time: 15 Minutes

Servings: 2-4

Ingredients:

- ½ lb salted and grated cod
- 3 cups boiled and squeezed potatoes
- 1 tbsp. of wheat flour
- Salt and black pepper to taste

- 3 eggs
- 2 tbsp. chopped green aroma

Directions:

1. In a bowl, mix all the ingredients well.

2. Form the balls with your hands.

3. Fry in the air fryer at 4000F for 30 minutes or until golden brown.

93.Lobster Bang Bang

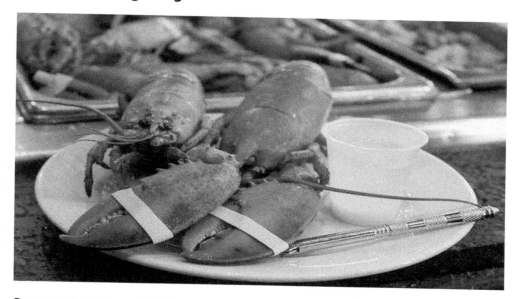

Preparation Time: 15 Minutes

Cooking Time: 20 Minutes

Servings: 4

Ingredients:

- 1 cup cornstarch
- ¼ teaspoon Sriracha powder
- ¼ cup mayonnaise
- ¼ cup sweet chili sauce
- 4 lbs Lobsters

Directions:

1. In a big bowl, combine corn-starch and Sriracha powder.
2. Dredge lobsters with this mixture.
3. Place lobsters in the air fryer.
4. Choose an air fry setting.

5. Cook at 400 degrees F for 7 minutes per side.

6. Mix the mayo and chili sauce.

7. Serve shrimp with sauce.

94.Honey Glazed Salmon

Preparation Time: 10 Minutes

Cooking Time: 35 Minutes

Servings: 1

Ingredients:

- ¼ cup soy sauce
- ½ cup honey
- 1 tablespoon lemon juice
- 1 oz. orange juice
- 1 tablespoon brown sugar
- 1 teaspoon olive oil
- 1 tablespoon red wine vinegar
- 1 scallion, chopped
- 1 clove garlic, minced
- Salt and pepper to taste
- 1 salmon fillet

Directions:

1. Mix all the ingredients except salt, pepper and salmon.

2. Place mixture in a pan over medium heat.

3. Bring to a boil.

4. Reduce heat.

5. Simmer for 15 minutes.

6. Turn off heat and transfer sauce to a bowl.

7. Sprinkle salt and pepper on both sides of the salmon.

8. Add salmon to the air fryer.

9. Select grill function.

95.Crispy Fish Fillet
Preparation Time: 10 Minutes

Cooking Time: 30 Minutes

Servings: 2

Ingredients:

- 2 cod fillets
- 1 teaspoon Old Bay seasoning
- Salt and pepper to taste
- ½ cup all-purpose flour
- 1 egg, beaten
- 2 cups breadcrumbs

Directions:

1. Sprinkle both sides of cod with Old Bay seasoning, salt and pepper.

2. Coat with flour, dip in egg and dredge with breadcrumbs.

3. Add fish to the air fryer.

4. Select air fry setting.

5. Cook at 400 degrees F for 5 to 6 minutes per side.

96.Garlic Butter Lobster Tails
Preparation Time: 10 Minutes

Cooking Time: 15 Minutes

Servings: 2

Ingredients:

- 2 lobster tails
- 2 cloves garlic, minced
- 2 tablespoons butter

- 1 teaspoon lemon juice
- 1 teaspoon chopped chives
- Salt to taste

Directions:

1. Butterfly the lobster tails.

2. Place the meat on top of the shell.

3. Mix the remaining ingredients in a bowl.

4. Add lobster tails inside the air fryer.

5. Set it to air fry.

6. Spread garlic butter on the meat.

7. Cook at 380 degrees F for 5 minutes.

8. Spread more butter on top.

9. Cook for another 2 to 3 minutes.

97.Pesto Fish

Preparation Time: 10 Minutes

Cooking Time: 15 Minutes

Servings: 4

Ingredients:

- 1 tablespoon olive oil
- 4 fish fillets
- Salt and pepper to taste
- 1 cup olive oil
- 3 cloves garlic
- 1 ½ cups fresh basil leaves
- 2 tablespoons Parmesan cheese, grated
- 3 tablespoons pine nuts

Directions:

1. Drizzle olive oil over fish fillets and season with salt and pepper.

2. Add remaining ingredients to a food processor.

3. Pulse until smooth.

4. Transfer pesto to a bowl and set aside.

5. Add fish to the air fryer.

6. Select grill setting.

7. Cook at 320 degrees F for 5 minutes per side.

8. Spread pesto on top of the fish before serving.

98.Mozzarella Spinach Quiche

Prep time: 10 min

Cook time: 45 min

Yield: 6 servings

Ingredients:

- 4 eggs
- 10 oz. frozen spinach, thawed
- 1/2 cup mozzarella cheese, shredded
- 1/4 cup parmesan cheese, grated
- 8 oz. mushrooms, sliced
- 2 oz. feta cheese, crumbled
- 1 cup almond milk
- 1 garlic clove, minced
- Pepper
- Salt

Directions:

24. Spray a pie dish with cooking spray and set it aside.

25. Insert wire rack in rack position 6. Select bake, set temperature 350 f, timer for 45 minutes. Press start to preheat the oven.

26. Spray medium pan with cooking spray and heat over medium heat.

27. Add garlic, mushrooms, pepper, and salt in a pan and sauté for 5 minutes.

28. Add spinach to the pie dish, then add sautéed mushroom on top of spinach.

29. Sprinkle feta cheese over spinach and mushroom.

30. In a bowl, whisk eggs, parmesan cheese, and almond milk.

31. Pour egg mixture over spinach and mushroom, then sprinkle shredded mozzarella cheese and bake for 45 minutes.

32. Sliced and serve.

99.Cheesy Zucchini Quiche

Total time: 1 hour 10 min

Prep time: 10 min

Cook time: 60 min

Yield: 8 servings

Ingredients:

- 2 eggs
- 2 cups cheddar cheese, shredded
- 1 1/2 cup almond milk
- Pepper
- Salt
- 2 lbs. zucchini, sliced

Directions:

1. Set aside and oil the quiche pan with cooking oil.

2. Wire rack insertion at rack position 6. Pick bake, set temperature to 375 f, 60-minute timer. To preheat the oven, press start.

3. With pepper and salt, season the zucchini and set aside for 30 minutes.

4. Mix the almond milk, spice, and salt with the eggs in a big cup.

5. Stir well and Mix sliced cheddar cheese.

6. Arrange slices of zucchini in a plate of quiche.

7. Pour the combination of eggs over the slices of zucchini and scatter with shredded cheese. For 60 minutes, roast.

8. Enjoy and serve.

100.Healthy Asparagus Quiche

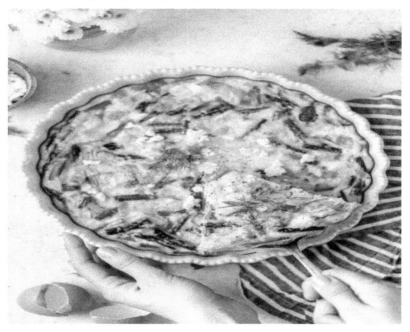

Total time: 1 hour 10 min

Prep time: 10 min

Cook time: 60 min

Yield: 6 servings

Ingredients:

- 5 eggs, beaten
- 1 cup almond milk
- 15 asparagus spears, cut ends then cut asparagus in half
- 1 cup Swiss cheese, shredded
- 1/4 tsp. thyme
- 1/4 tsp. white pepper
- 1/4 tsp. salt

Directions:

Grease quiche pan with cooking spray and set aside.

Insert wire rack in rack position 6. Select bake, set temperature 350 f, timer for 60 minutes. Press start to preheat the oven.

In a bowl, whisk together eggs, thyme, white pepper, almond milk, and salt.

Arrange asparagus in quiche pan, then pour egg mixture over asparagus. Sprinkle with shredded cheese.

Bake for 60 minutes.

Sliced and serve.

Conclusion

Before you know how to use an Air Fryer, you need to make some plans before using it and take some steps accordingly. Such as getting an amazing recipe book to cook your food using an air fryer. This book will surely help you with that as it has covered a delicious range of air fryer recipes.

KETO DIET FOR WOMEN OVER 50

The Complete Ketogenic Diet Step by Step To Learn How to Easily Lose Weight for Woman

By Jason Smith

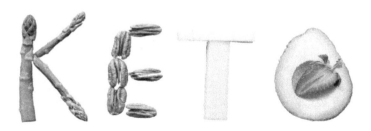

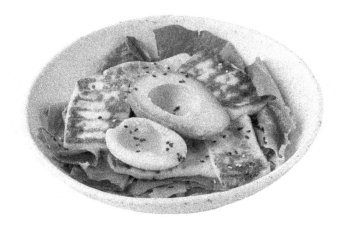

information is without a contract or any type of guarantee assurance.

The trademarks used are without any consent, and the publication of the trademark is without permission or backing by the trademark owner. All trademarks and brands within this book are for clarifying purposes only and are owned by the owners themselves, not affiliated with this document.

Introduction

The keto diet is a diet that has higher and lower fat values. It decreases glucose & insulin levels and changes the body's digestion away from carbohydrates and more towards fat & ketones. A word used in a low-carb diet is "Ketogenic." The concept is to provide more calories from fat and protein and few from sugars. The consumption of a high, low-sugar diet, adequate-protein, is used in medicine to achieve difficult (unstable) epilepsy control in young people. Instead of sugar, the diet allows the body to eat fats. Usually, the nutritious starches are converted to sugar, which will then be distributed throughout the body and is particularly important in filling the mind's work. Keto diet can cause enormous declines in the levels of glucose and insulin.

How food affects your body

Our metabolic procedures survive if we do not get the right details, and our well-being declines. We can get overweight, malnourished, and at risk for the worsening of diseases and disorders, such as inflammatory disease, diabetes, and cardiovascular disease if women get an unhealthy amount of essential nutrients or nourishment that provides their body with inadequate guidance. The dietary supplements allow the cells in our bodies to serve their essential capacities. This quote from a well-known workbook shows how dietary supplements are important for our physical work. Supplements are the nourishment feed substances necessary for the growth, development, and support of the body's capacities. Fundamental claimed that when a supplement is absent, capability sections and thus decrease in human health. The metabolic processes are delayed when the intake of supplements usually may not fulfill the cell activity's supplement requirements.

The keto diet involves keeping to a relatively low-carb, high-fat diet to put the body into a physiological state called ketosis. This makes fat intake increasingly productive for the health. When starting the diet, the ketogenic diet can induce a decrease in the drive, as the dieter will suffer side effects of carb removal and possibly low carb influenza. Whenever the detox and influenza-like symptoms have gone, and the dieter has transitioned to the reduced way of living, leading to weight loss from the diet, the charisma would in all likelihood reset and probably be comparable to earlier. Although the drive alert has a lot of credibility in the mainstream, in other words, supplementation provides advice to our bodies on how to function. In this sense, nourishment can be seen as a source of "information for the body." Pondering food along these lines gives one a view of the nourishment beyond calories or grams, fantastic food sources, or bad food sources. Instead of avoiding food sources, this perspective pushes us to reflect on the nutrients we can add. Instead of reviewing nourishment as the enemy, we look at nourishment to reduce health and disease by having the body look after ability.

Kidney and Heart Disease

When the body is low in electrolytes and fluid over the increased pee, electrolyte loss, such as magnesium, sodium, and potassium, can be caused. This will render people inclined to suffer serious kidney problems. Flushing out is not a joke and can lead to light-headedness, damage to the kidney, or kidney problems. Just like electrolytes are essential for the heart's standard stomping, this can place a dieter at the risk of cardiac arrhythmia. "Electrolyte appears to lack are not joking, and that may bring in an irregular heartbeat, that can be harmful,"

Yo-yo Dieting designs

When individuals encounter difficulties staying on the prohibitive diet indefinitely, the keto diet will also cause yo-yo dieting. That can have other adverse effects on the body.

Other effects

Other responses can involve terrible breath, fatigue, obstruction, irregular menstrual periods, reduced bone density, and trouble with rest. For even the most part, other consequences are not so much considered since it is impossible to observe dieters on a long-term assumption to discover the food schedule's permanent effects.

Wholesome Concerns

"There is still a dread amongst healthcare professionals that certain high intakes of extremely unhealthy fats will have a longer journey negative effect," she explained. Weight loss will also, for the time being, complicate the data. As overweight people get in form, paying less attention to how they do so, they sometimes end up with much better lipid profiles and blood glucose levels.

In comparison, the keto diet is extremely low in particular natural ingredients, fruits, nuts, and veggies that are as nutritious as a whole. Without these supplements, fiber, some carbohydrates, minerals, including phytochemicals that come along with these nourishments, will move through people on a diet. In the long run, this has vital public health consequences, such as bone degradation and increased risk of infinite diseases.

Sodium

The mixture of sodium (salt), fat, sugar, including bunches of sodium, will make inexpensive food more delicious for many people. However, diets rich in sodium will trigger fluid retention, which is why you can feel puffy, bloated, or swelled up in the aftermath of consuming cheap food. For those with pulse problems, a diet rich in sodium is also harmful. Sodium can increase circulatory stress and add weight to the cardiovascular structure. If one survey reveals, about % of grown-ups lose how much salt is in their affordable food meals. The study looked at 993 adults and found that the initial prediction was often smaller than the actual figure (1,292 mg). This suggests the sodium gauges in the abundance of 1,000 mg is off. One affordable meal could be worth a significant proportion of your day.

Impact on the Respiratory Framework

An overabundance of calories can contribute to weight gain from cheap foods. This will add to the weight. Obesity creates the risk of respiratory conditions, including asthma with shortness of breath. The extra pounds can put pressure on the heart and lungs, and with little intervention, side effects can occur. When you walk, climb stairs, or work out, you can notice trouble breathing. For youngsters, the possibility of respiratory problems is especially obvious. One research showed that young people who consume cheap food at least three days a week are bound to develop asthma.

Impact on the focal sensory system

For the time being, cheap food may satisfy hunger; however, long-haul effects are more detrimental. Individuals who consume inexpensive food and processed bakery items are 51 percent bound to generate depression than people who do not eat or eat either of those foods.

Impact on the conceptive framework

The fixings in cheap food and lousy nourishment can affect your money. One analysis showed that phthalates are present in prepared nourishment. Phthalates are synthetic compounds that can mess with the way your body's hormones function. Introduction to substantial amounts of these synthetics, like birth absconds, could prompt regenerative problems.

Impact on the integumentary framework (skin, hair, nails)

The food you eat may affect your skin's appearance, but it's not going to be the food you imagine. The responsibility for skin dry out breakouts has traditionally been claimed by sweets and sticky nourishments such as pizza. Nevertheless, as per the Mayo Clinic, there are starches. Carb-rich foods cause glucose jumps, and these sudden leaps in glucose levels can induce inflammation of the skin. Additionally, as shown by one investigation, young people and young women who consume inexpensive food at any pace three days a week are expected to create skin inflammation. Dermatitis is a skin disease that causes dry, irritated skin spots that are exacerbated.

Impact on the skeletal framework (bones)

Acids in the mouth can be enlarged by carbohydrates and sugar in inexpensive food and treated food. These acids may distinguish tooth lacquer. Microorganisms can take hold when the tooth veneer disappears, and depressions can occur. Weight will also prompt issues with bone thickness and bulk. The more severe chance of falling and breaking bones is for heavy individuals. It is important to continue training, develop muscles that support the bones, and sustain a balanced diet to prevent bone loss. One investigation showed that the measure of calories, sugar, and sodium in cheap food meals remains, to a large degree, constant because of attempts to bring problems to light and make women more intelligent consumers. As women get busier and eat out more often, it could have antagonistic effects on women and America's healthcare structure.

Chapter 1: Keto Diet and Its Benefits

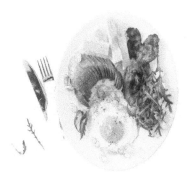

In the case of a ketogenic diet, the aim is to restrict carbohydrate intake to break down fat for power. When this occurs, to produce ketones that are by-products of the metabolism, the liver breaks down fat. These ketones are used in the absence of glucose to heat the body. A ketogenic diet takes the body into a "ketosis" mode. A metabolic condition that happens as ketone bodies in the blood contains most of the body's energy rather than glucose from carbohydrate-produced foods (such as grains, all sources of sugar or fruit). This compares with a glycolytic disorder, where blood glucose produces most of the body's power.

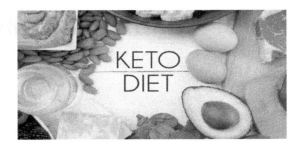

1.1. Keto Diet and its Success

The keto diet is successful in many studies, especially among obese men and women. The results suggest that KD can help manage situations such as:

- Obesity.
- Heart disease.

It is difficult to relate the ketogenic diet to cardiovascular disease risk factors. Several studies have shown that keto diets may contribute to substantial reductions in overall cholesterol, rises in levels of HDL cholesterol, decreases in levels of triglycerides and decreases in levels of LDL cholesterol, as well as possible changes in levels of blood pressure.

- Neurological disorders, including Alzheimer's, dementia, multiple sclerosis and Parkinson's.
- Polycystic ovarian syndrome (PCOS), among women of reproductive age, is the most prevalent endocrine condition.
- Certain forms of cancer, including cancers of the liver, colon, pancreas and ovaries.
- Diabetes Type 2. Among type 2 diabetics, it can also minimize the need for drugs.
- Seizure symptoms and seizures.
- And others.

1.2. Why Do the Ketogenic Diet

By exhausting the body from its sugar store, Ketogenic works to start sorting fat and protein for vitality, inducing ketosis (and weight loss).

1. Helps in weight loss

To convert fat into vitality, it takes more effort than it takes to turn carbohydrates into vitality. A ketogenic diet along these lines can help speed up weight loss. In comparison, because the diet is rich in protein, it doesn't leave you starving as most diets do. Five findings uncovered tremendous weight loss from a ketogenic diet in a meta-examination of 13 complex randomized controlled preliminaries.

2. Diminishes skin break out

There are different causes for the breakout of the skin, and food and glucose can be established. Eating a balanced diet of prepared and refined sugars can alter gut microorganisms and emphasize sensational variances in glucose, both of which would affect the skin's health. Therefore, that is anything but surprising that a keto diet may reduce a few instances of skin inflammation by decreasing carb entry.

3. May help diminish the danger of malignancy

There has been a lot of study on the ketogenic diet and how it could effectively forestall or even cure those malignant growths. One investigation showed that the ketogenic diet might be a corresponding effective treatment with chemotherapy and radiation in people with malignancy. It is because it can cause more oxidative concern than in ordinary cells in malignancy cells.

Some hypotheses indicate that it may decrease insulin entanglements, which could be linked to some cancers because the ketogenic diet lowers elevated glucose.

4. Improves heart health

There is some indication that the diet will boost cardiac health by lowering cholesterol by accessing the ketogenic diet in a balanced manner (which looks at avocados as a healthy fat rather than pork skins). One research showed that LDL ("Terrible") cholesterol levels fundamentally expanded among those adopting the keto diet. In turn, the LDL ("terrible") cholesterol fell.

5. May secure mind working

More study into the ketogenic diet and even the mind is needed. A few studies indicate that the keto diet has Neuro-protective effects. These can help treat or curtail Parkinson's, Alzheimer's, and even some rest problems. One research also showed that young people had increased and psychological work during a ketogenic diet.

6. Possibly lessens seizures

The theory that the combination of fat, protein, and carbohydrates modifies how vitality is utilized by the body, inducing ketosis. Ketosis is an abnormal level of Ketone in the blood. In people with epilepsy, ketosis will prompt a reduction in seizures.

7. Improves health in women with PCOS

An endocrine condition that induces augmented ovaries with pimples is polycystic ovarian disorder PCOS). On the opposite, a high-sugar diet can affect those with PCOS. On the ketogenic diet and PCOS, there are not many clinical tests. One pilot study involving five women on 24 weeks showed that the ketogenic diet:

- Aided hormone balance
- Improved luteinizing hormone (ILH)/follicle-invigorating hormone (FSH) proportions
- Increased weight loss
- Improved fasting insulin

For children who suffer the adverse effects of a particular problem (such as Lennox-gastaut disease or Rett disorder) and do not respond to seizure prescription, keto is also prescribed as suggested by the epilepsy foundation.

They note that the number of seizures these children had can be greatly reduced by keto, with 10 to 15 percent turns out to be sans seizure. It may also help patients to reduce the portion of their prescription in some circumstances. Be it as it can, the ketogenic diet still many effective trials to back up its advantages. For adults with epilepsy, the keto diet can likewise be helpful. It was considered as preferable to other diets in supporting people with:

- Epilepsy
- Type 2 diabetes
- Type 1 diabetes
- High blood pressure
- Heart disease
- Polycystic ovary syndrome
- Fatty liver disease
- Cancer
- Migraines

- Alzheimer's infection
- Parkinson's infection
- Chronic inflammation
- High blood sugar levels
- Obesity

The ketogenic diet will be beneficial, regardless of whether you are not in danger from any of these disorders. A portion of the advantages that are enjoyed by the vast majority are:

- An increment in vitality
- Improved body arrangement
- Better cerebrum work
- A decline in aggravation

As should be clear, the ketogenic diet has a vast variety of advantages, but is it preferable to other diets?

8. Treating epilepsy — the origins of the ketogenic diet

Until sometime in 1998, the major analysis on epilepsy and the keto diets was not distributed. Of about 150 children, almost each of whom had several seizures a week, despite taking two psychosis drugs in either situation. The children were given a one-year initial ketogenic diet. Around 34 percent of infants, or slightly more than 33 percent, had a 90 percent decline in seizures after three months.

The healthy diet was claimed to be "more feasible than just a substantial lot of new anticonvulsant medications and is much endured by families and kids when it is effective." Not only was the keto diet supportive. It was, however, more useful than other drugs usually used.

9. Improving blood pressure with the ketogenic diet

A low-sugar intake is more effective at reducing the pulse than just a low-fat or moderate-fat diet. Restricting starches often provides preferable results over the mix of a low-fat regimen and a relaxing weight-loss/pulse.

10. The power to improve Alzheimer's disease

Alzheimer's disease patients also agree with organic chemistry." high sugar acceptance deepens academic performance in patient populations with Alzheimer's infectious disease." It means that more starches are consumed in the cerebrum. Will the reverse (trying to eat fewer carbs) improve the functioning of the cerebrum?

Other mental health benefits that ketone bodies have:

- They forestall neuronal loss.
- They ensure synapses against various sorts of damage.
- They save neuron work.

1.3. The Benefits of Ketogenic Diet

The board provides many substantial advantages when choosing a ketogenic diet for diabetes. Living in a stable ketosis state causes a tremendous change in blood glucose regulation and weight loss. Other frequent advantages provided include:

- Improvements in insulin affectability
- Lower circulatory strain
- Usually enhancements in cholesterol levels.
- Reduced reliance on taking drugs

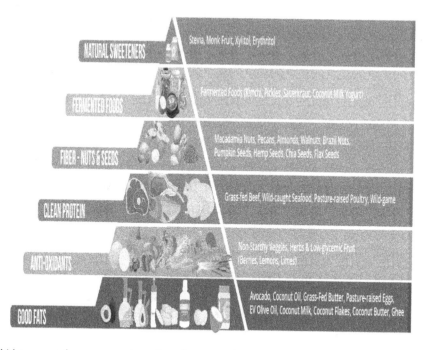

We send you a short science behind the ketogenic diet in this book and how it attempts to give these particular benefits.

1. Weight loss and support

The ketogenic diet's significant benefit is achieving accelerated weight loss, reducing starches necessary to be in a ketosis state, causing both a noteworthy decrease in muscle vs. fats and bulk increase and maintenance. Studies have shown that a low-carb, keto diet can produce an all-inclusive duration of solid weight loss. For one year, a big person had the opportunity to lose, by and large, 15 kilograms. It was 3 kg, which is more than the low-fat food used in the study carried out.

2. Blood glucose control

The other main reason for maintaining a ketogenic diet for people with diabetes is its ability to reduce and regulate glucose levels. The substitute (macronutrient) that improves glucose the most is starch. Since the keto diet is low in starch, the greater rises in glucose are dispensed with. Ketogenic diets prove that they are effective in reducing hba1c, a long-term blood glucose regulation percentage. A natural decrease of 17 mmol/mol (1.5 percent) in hba1c levels for persons with type 2 diabetes. People with other forms of diabetes, such as diabetes and LADA, can also expect to see a strong decline in glucose levels and increase control. Remember that if an increase in blood glucose regulation is sustained over different years, this will reduce intricacies. It is necessary to play it safe for those on insulin, or otherwise at risk of hypos, to avoid the incidence of hypos.

Decreasing drug reliance on diabetes. Since it is so effective at lowering glucose levels, the keto diet provides the added benefit of allowing people with type 2 diabetes to decrease their dependency on diabetes medication.

Persons on insulin and other hypertension prescriptions (Sulphonylureas & Glinides, for example) may need to reduce their portions before initiating a ketogenic diet to avoid hypotension. For advice on this, contact your primary care provider.

3. Insulin affectability

To further restore insulin affectability, a ketogenic diet has emerged since it dispenses with the root driver of insulin obstruction, which is too high insulin levels in the bloodstream. This diet advances supported periods with low insulin since low carbohydrate levels indicate lower insulin levels. A high diet of starch resembles putting petroleum on the insulin obstruction fire. A more influential need for insulin is indicated by elevated sugar, and this aggravates insulin opposition. A ketogenic diet, by correlation, turns down insulin levels since fat is the least insulin-requiring macronutrient. In comparison, bringing the insulin levels down also helps with fat intake, provided that elevated insulin levels inhibit fat breakdown. The body will differentiate fat cells at the point that insulin levels decrease for several hours.

4. Hypertension control

It is estimated that 16 million people in the U.K. suffer from hypertension. Hypertension, for example, cardiovascular disease, stroke, and renal disease, is related to the scope of health disorders. Different studies have demonstrated that a ketogenic diet can reduce circulatory stress levels in overweight or type 2 diabetes people. It is also a part of metabolic imbalance.

5. Cholesterol levels

For the most part, ketogenic diets bring in reductions in cholesterol levels. LDL cholesterol levels are usually reduced, and HDL cholesterol levels increase, which is healthy. The amount of absolute cholesterol to HDL is possibly the most substantiated proportion of safe cholesterol. It can be effectively detected by taking the full cholesterol result and partitioning it by your HDLS result. It indicates good cholesterol, on the off chance that the amount you get is 3.5 or lower. Study findings suggest that ketogenic diets are normally possible to increase this proportion of good cholesterol.

After starting a ketogenic, a few individuals can display an expansion in LDL and all-out cholesterol. It is generally taken as a bad indicator, but this does not speak of compounding in heart health if the absolute cholesterol to HDL ratio is appropriate.

Cholesterol is a confounding topic, and if your cholesterol levels essentially shift on a ketogenic diet, your PCP is the optimization technique of exhortation. More simple mental results. Other typically announced advantages of eating a ketogenic diet are emotional insight, an increased capacity to center, and superior memory. Expanding the admission of omega-3 healthy fats, such as those present in slick fish such as salmon, fish, and mackerel, will boost the state of mind and the ability to read. It is because omega-3 extends an unsaturated fat called DHAS, which makes up 15 to 30 percent of the cerebrum of females. The discovery of beta-hydroxybutyrate, a type of Ketone, allows for long-term memory work to be facilitated.

6. Satiety

The effects of ketogenic diets impact malnutrition. As the body responds to being in a ketosis state, it becomes acclimatized to obtain vitality from muscle to fat ratio differentiation, which will alleviate appetite and desires.

They are possible at:

- **Reducing desires**
- **Reducing inclination for sugary nourishments**
- **Helping you feel full for more**

Weight loss will also reduce leptin levels attributable to a ketogenic diet, which will increase the affectability of leptin and thus gain satiety.

1.4. Keto Shopping List

A keto diet meal schedule for women above 5o+ years and a menu that will transform the body. Generally speaking, the keto diet is low in carbohydrates, high in fat and moderate in protein. While adopting a ketogenic diet, carbs are routinely reduced to under 50 grams every day, but stricter and looser adaptations of the diet exist.

• Proteins can symbolize about 20 percent of strength requirements, whereas carbohydrates are usually restricted to 5 percent.

• The body retains its fat for the body to use as energy production.

Most of the cut carbs should be supplanted by fats and convey about 75% of your all-out caloric intake.

The body processes ketones while it is in ketosis, particles released from cholesterol in the blood glucose is low, as yet another source of energy.

Because fat is always kept a strategic distance from its unhealthy content, research demonstrates that the keto diet is essentially better than low-fat diets to advance weight reduction.

In contrast, keto diets minimize desire and improve satiation, which is especially useful when getting in shape.

Fatty cuts of PROTEIN: *Keto Diet Shopping list*

1. GROUND BEEF - RIBEYE STEAK
2. PORK BELLY ROAST +BACON
3. BEEF OR PORK SAUSAGE
4. WILD CAUGHT SALMON
5. SARDINES OR TUNA
6. CHICKEN THIGHS OR LEGS
7. TURKEY LEGS
8. DEER STEAKS
9. EGGS
10. DUCK EGGS
11.

FATS:
1. BUTTER
2. OLIVE OIL
3. COCONUT OIL
4. COCONUT BUTTER
5. MCT OIL
6. AVOCADO
7. GHEE
8. BACON GREASE
9. AVOCADO OIL

Green Leafy VEGGIES:
1. BROCCOLI
2. CAULIFLOWER
3. GREEN BEANS
4. BRUSSEL SPROUTS
5. KALE
6. SPINACH
7. CHARD
8. CABBAGE
9. BOK CHOY
10. CELERY
11. ARUGULA
12. ASPARAGUS
13. ZUCCHINI
14. YELLOW SQUASH
15. MUSHROOMS
16. OLIVES
17. ARTICHOKE
18. CUCUMBERS
19. ONIONS
20. GARLIC
21. OKRA

NUTS AND SEEDS:
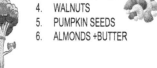
1. MACADAMIA NUTS+BUTTER
2. BRAZIL NUTS+BUTTER
3. PECANS+BUTTER
4. WALNUTS
5. PUMPKIN SEEDS
6. ALMONDS +BUTTER

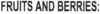

FRUITS AND BERRIES:
1. POMEGRANATE
2. GRAPEFRUIT
3. BLUEBERRIES
4. RASPBERRIES
5. LEMON
6. LIME
7. AVOCADO

MUST HAVE MISCELLANEOUS:
1. ALMOND+COCONUT FLOUR
2. COCONUT BUTTER
3. 85% DARK CHOCOLATE
4. PORK RINDS
5. COCONUT CREAM
6. COCONUT FLAKES

1.5. Keto-Friendly Foods to Eat

Meals and bites should be based on the accompanying nourishment when following a ketogenic diet:

Eggs: pastured eggs are the best choice for all-natural eggs.

Meat: hamburger grass- nourished, venison, pork, organ meat, and buffalo.

Full-fat dairy: yogurt, cream and margarine.

Full-fat Cheddar: Cheddar, mozzarella, brie, cheddar goat and cheddar cream.

Nuts and seeds: almonds, pecans, macadamia nuts, peanuts, pumpkin seeds, and flaxseeds.

Poultry: turkey and chicken.

Fatty fish: Wild-got salmon, herring, and mackerel

Nut margarine: Natural nut, almond, and cashew spreads.

Vegetables that are not boring: greens, broccoli, onions, mushrooms, and peppers.

Condiments: salt, pepper, lemon juice, vinegar, flavors and crisp herbs.

Fats: coconut oil, olive oil, coconut margarine, avocado oil, and sesame oil.

Avocados: it is possible to add whole avocados to practically any feast or bite.

1.6. Nourishments to avoid

Although adopting a keto diet, keep away from carbohydrate-rich nutrients.

It is important to restrict the accompanying nourishments:

- **Sweetened beverages:** beer, juice, better teas, and drinks for sports.
- **Pasta:** noodles and spaghetti.
- **Grains and vegetable articles:** maize, rice, peas, oats for breakfast
- **Starchy vegetables:** Butternut squash, Potatoes, beans, sweet potatoes, pumpkin and peas.
- **Beans and vegetables:** chickpeas, black beans, kidney beans and lentils.
- **Fruit:** citrus, apples, pineapple and bananas.
- **Sauces containing high-carbohydrates:** BBQ' sauce, a sugar dressing with mixed greens, and dipping's.
- **Hot and bread items:** white bread, whole wheat bread, wafers, cookies, doughnuts, rolls, etc.
- **Sweets and sweet foods:** honey, ice milk, candy, chocolate syrup, agave syrup, coconut sugar.
- **Blended refreshments:** Sugar-blended cocktails and beer.

About the assumption that carbs should be small, low-glycemic organic goods, for example, when a keto-macronutrient is served, spread, berries may be satisfied with restricted quantities. Be sure to choose safe sources of protein and eliminate prepared sources of food and bad fats.

It is worth keeping the accompanying stuff away from:

1. Diet nutrients: Foods containing counterfeit hues, contaminants and carbohydrates, such as aspartame and sugar alcohols.

2. Unhealthy fats: Such as corn and canola oil, include shortening, margarine, and cooking oils.

3. Processed foods: Fast foods, bundled food sources, and frozen meats, such as wieners and meats for lunch.

1.8. One week Keto Diet Plan

(Day 1): Monday

Breakfast: Eggs fried in seasoned butter served over vegetables.

Lunch: A burger of grass-bolstered with avocado, mushrooms, and cheddar on a tray of vegetables.

Dinner: Pork chops and French beans sautéed in vegetable oil.

(Day 2): Tuesday

Breakfast: Omelet of mushroom.

Lunch: Salmon, blended vegetables, tomato, and celery on greens.

Dinner: Roast chicken and sautéed cauliflower.

(Day 3): Wednesday

Breakfast: Cheddar cheese, eggs, and bell peppers.

Lunch: Blended veggies with hard-bubbled eggs, avocado, turkey, and cheddar.

Dinner: Fried salmon sautéed in coconut oil.

(Day 4): Thursday

Breakfast: Granola with bested full-fat yogurt.

Lunch: Steak bowl of cheddar, cauliflower rice, basil, avocado, as well as salsa.

Dinner: Bison steak and mushy cauliflower.

(Day 5): Friday

Breakfast: Pontoons of Avocado egg (baked).

Lunch: Chicken served with Caesar salad.

Dinner: Pork, with veggies.

(Day 6): Saturday

Breakfast: Avocado and cheddar with cauliflower.

Lunch: Bunless burgers of salmon.

Dinner: Parmesan cheddar with noodles topped with meatballs.

(Day 7): Sunday

Breakfast: Almond Milk, pecans and Chia pudding.

Lunch: Cobb salad made of vegetables, hard-boiled eggs, mango, cheddar, and turkey.

Dinner: Curry chicken.

Chapter 2: Health Concerns for Women Over 50+

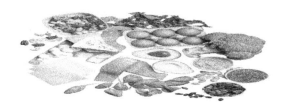

This chapter will give you a detailed view of the health concerns for women over 50.

2.1. Menopause

Healthy maturation includes large propensities such as eating healthy, avoiding regular prescription mistakes, monitoring health conditions, receiving suggested screenings, or being dynamic. Getting more seasoned involves change, both negative and positive, but you can admire maturing on the off chance of understanding your body's new things and finding a way to maintain your health. As you age, a wide range of things happens to your body. Unexpectedly, your skin, bones, and even cerebrum may start to carry on. Try not to let the advances that accompany adulthood get you off guard.

Here's a segment of the normal ones:

1. The Bones: In mature age, bones may become slender and progressively weaker, especially in women, leading to the delicate bone disease known as osteoporosis once in a while. Diminishing bones and decreasing bone mass can put you at risk for falls that can occur in broken bones without much of a stretch result. Make sure you talk to your doctor about what you can do to prevent falls and osteoporosis.

2. The Heart: While a healthy diet and normal exercise can keep your heart healthy, it may turn out to be somewhat amplified, lowering your pulse and thickening the heart dividers.

3. The Sensory system and Mind: It can trigger changes in your reflexes and even your skills by becoming more seasoned. While dementia is certainly not an ordinary outcome of mature age, individuals must encounter some slight memory loss as they become more stated. The formation of plaques and tangles, abnormalities that could ultimately lead to dementia, can harm cells in the cerebrum and nerves.

4. The Stomach: A structure associated with your stomach. As you age, it turns out that your stomach-related is all the more firm and inflexible and does not contract as often. For example, stomach torment, obstruction, and feelings of nausea can prompt problems with this change; a superior diet can help.

5. The Abilities: You can see that your hearing and vision is not as good as it ever was. Maybe you'll start losing your sense of taste. Flavors might not appear as unique to you. Your odor and expertise in touch can also weaken. In order to respond, the body requires more time and needs more to revitalize it.

6. The Teeth: Throughout the years, the intense veneer protecting your teeth from rot will begin to erode, making you exposed to pits. Likewise, gum injury is a problem for more developed adults. Your teeth and gums will

guarantee great dental cleanliness. Dry mouth, which is a common symptom of seniors' multiple drugs, can also be a concern.

7. The Skin: Your skin loses its versatility at a mature age and can tend to droop and wrinkle. Nonetheless, the more you covered your skin when you were younger from sun exposure and smoke, the healthier your skin would look as you get more mature. Start securing your skin right now to prevent more injury, much like skin malignancy.

8. The Sexual Conviviality: When the monthly period ends following menopause, many women undergo physical changes such as vaginal oil loss. Men can endure erectile brokenness. Fortunately, it is possible to handle the two problems successfully.

A normal part of maturing is a series of substantial improvements, but they don't need to back you up. Furthermore, you should do a lot to protect your body and keep it as stable as you would imagine, given the circumstances.

2.2. Keys to Aging Well

Although good maturation must preserve your physical fitness, it is also vital to appreciate the maturity and growth you acquire with propelling years. Its fine to rehearse healthy propensities for an extraordinary period, but it's never beyond the point of no return to gain the benefits of taking great account of yourself, even as you get more developed.

Here are some healthy maturing tips at every point of life that are a word of wisdom:

- Keep dynamic physically with a normal workout.
- With loved ones and inside your locale, remain socially diverse.
- Eat a balanced, well-adjusted diet, dumping low-quality food to intake low-fat, fiber-rich, and low-cholesterol.
- Do not forget yourself: daily enrollment at this stage with your primary care provider, dental surgeon, and optometrist is becoming increasingly relevant.
- Taking all medications as the primary care provider coordinates.
- Limit the consumption of liquor and break off smoke.
- Receive the rest your body wants.

Finally, it is necessary to deal with your physical self for a long time, but it is vital that you still have an eye on your passionate health. Receive and enjoy the rewards of your long life every single day. It is the perfect chance to enjoy better health and pleasure.

1. Eat a healthy diet

For more developed development, excellent nourishment and sanitation are especially critical. You need to regularly ensure that you eat a balanced, tailored diet. To help you decide on astute diet options and practice healthy nutrition, follow these guidelines.

2. Stay away from common medication mistakes

Drugs can cure health conditions and allow you to continue to lead a long, stable life. Drugs may also cause real health problems at the stage that they are misused. To help you decide on keen decisions about the remedy and over-the-counter medications you take, use these assets.

3. Oversee health conditions

Working with your healthcare provider to monitor health issues such as diabetes, osteoporosis, and hypertension is important. To treat these regular health problems, you need to get familiar with the medications and gadgets used.

4. Get screened

Health scans are an effective means of helping to perceive health conditions - even before any signs or side effects are given. Tell the healthcare provider what direct health scans are for you to determine how much you can be screened.

5. Be active

Exercise, as well as physical action, can help you to remain solid and fit. You just don't have to go to an exercise center. Converse about proper ways that you really can be dynamic with your healthcare professional. Look at the assets of the FDA and our accomplices in the administration.

2.3. Skin Sagging

There are also ways to prevent age from sagging, which are:

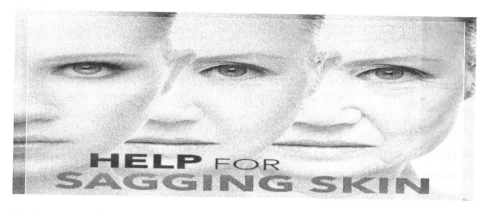

1. Unassuming Fixing and Lifting

These systems are called non-obtrusive methodologies of non-intrusive skin fixing on the basis that they leave your skin unblemished. A while later, you won't have a cut injury, a cut, or crude skin. You may see and grow some impermanent redness, but that is usually the main sign that you have a technique.

It is what you can expect from a skin-fixing method that is non-intrusive:

- **Results:** seem to come step by step, so they seem normal to be

- **Downtime:** zero to little

- **Colorblind:** secure for people with all skin hues

- **Body-wide use:** you can patch the skin almost anywhere on your body.

**Ultrasonic dermatologists use ultrasound to transmit heat deep into the tissue.**

Key concern: warming will induce more collagen to be created by your body. Many individuals see the unobtrusive raising and fixing within two and a half years of one procedure. By getting additional drugs, you can get more benefits.

**During this procedure, the dermatologist places a radiofrequency device on the skin that warms the tissue beneath.**

Key concern: Most people get one treatment and instantly feel an obsession. Your body needs some money to manufacture collagen, so you'll see the best effects in about half a year. By getting more than one treatment, a few persons benefit.

**Some lasers will send heat deeply through the skin without injuring the skin's top layer by laser therapy. These lasers are used to repair skin everywhere and can be especially effective for fixing free skin on the tummy and upper arms.**

Primary concern: to get outcomes, you may need 3 to 5 drugs, which occur step by step somewhere in the region of 2 and a half years after the last procedure.

2. Most fixing and lifting without medical procedure

While these methodologies will deliver you increasingly measurable results, considering all, they will not give you the aftereffects of an operation such as a facelift, eyelid surgical treatment, or neck lift, insignificantly pleasing to the eye skin fixing techniques. Negligibly obtrusive skin fixing requires less personal time than surgical treatment, however. It also conveys less chance of reactions.

3. How to look younger than your age without Botox, lasers and surgery, plus natural remedies for skin sagging

It is possible to become more experienced in this lifetime. However, you don't need to look at your age on the off chance you'd like not to. Truth be told, if you have been wondering how you would look as youthful as you feel, we will be eager to bet that you feel a lot more youthful than the amount you call your "age!"

2.4. Weight loss

Quality preparation builds the quality of your muscles and improves your versatility.

Even though cardio is very important for lung health and the heart, getting more fit and keeping it off is anything but an incredible technique.

The weight will return quickly at the point when you quit doing a lot of cardio. An unquestionable requirement has cardio as a component of your general wellness routine; be that as it may, when you start going to the exercise centre, quality preparation should be the primary factor. Quality preparation increases your muscle's quality, but this will enhance your portability and the main thing known to build bone thickness (alongside appropriate supplements).

Weight-bearing exercises help build and maintain bulk and build bone quality and reduce the risk of osteoporosis. Many people over [the age of] 50 will stop regularly practicing due to torment in their joints or back or damage, but do not surrender. In any case, understand that because of age-related illness, hormone changes, and even social variables such as a busy life, it may seem more enthusiastic to pick up muscle as you age. As he would like to think that to build durable muscles, cardio will consume off fat and pick substantial weights with few representatives or lighter weights. Similarly, for generally speaking health and quality, remember exercise and diet are linked to the hip, likewise, as the trick of the year. ! Locate a professional who can help you get back into the groove and expect to get 2 hrs.

Thirty minutes of physical movement in any case [in] seven days to help to maintain your bulk and weight.

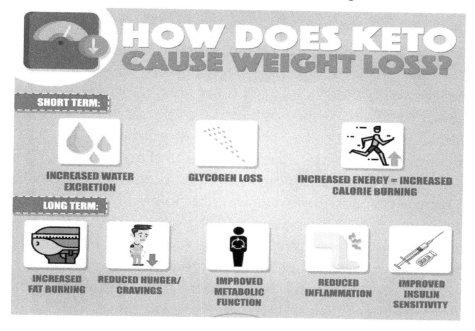

1. Try not to skip meals.

Testosterone and Estrogen decline gradually after some time, which also prompts fat collection because the body does not prepare sugar. We alternatively keep losing more bulk as we get older; this will cause our bodies' metabolic needs to lessen. Be that as it may, meal skipping can make you lack significant key medications required as we age, for example, by before large protein and calories. Tracking your energy levels throughout the day and obtaining sufficient calories/protein would also help you feel better on the scale, explaining how you will be burning more calories but less inefficiently. We also lose more bulk as we age, causing our metabolic rate to decrease. Be that as it may, skipping meals can make you lack important key supplements required as we age, for example, by an aging, metabolic rate.

2. Ensure you are getting enough rest.

"Perhaps the highest argument of over 50 years is a lack of rest," Amselem notes. Basically, rest may interfere with an important medical procedure, causing metabolic breakage in the system, in which the body turns weakness into hunger, urging you to eat. I plan to rest for seven to eight hours and, if necessary, take low rest. Rest is vital to a healthy weight because two hormones, leptin, and Ghrelin are released during rest, and they conclude a significant job in eating guidelines.

3. Relinquish old "rules" about weight loss and develop an outlook on health.

For the two women and men, age impacts weight loss, and that is on the basis that digestion backs off, hormone levels decay, in addition to there is a loss of bulk," "Nevertheless, that does not imply that mission is inconceivable to get more fit over age 50. Everybody else has to take a half hour's exercise, but there are two big reasons why it can't be done: you eat too much, or you are not active enough. The wellness movement encourages people to be aware of their own health, body and well-being. Being over 50 years old is not the end of the world. In fact, there is still a chance for us to live the rest of our lives as retirees. It is important to eat well, exercise, not smoke, and limit alcohol consumption in our lives. Our bodies are naturally aging, but we do not yet have to quit. Instead of falling prey to craze diets, make ongoing acclimatization to advance adjusted eating, and help yourself remember the benefits of exercise for your heart, stomach-related tract, and psychological well-being, despite the executives' weight.

2.5. Factors Influencing Fuel Utilization

The amount of each element in one's blood plasma determines the combination of fuels in the body. According to the researchers, the main element that determines how much of each nutrient is absorbed is the quantity of each nutrient eaten first by the body. The second considerations to take into account when assessing one's health is the amounts of hormones like insulin and glucagon, which must be in balance with one's diet. The third is the body's physical accumulation (cellular) of any nutrient, such as fat, muscle, and liver glycogen. Finally, the quantities of regulatory enzymes for glucose & fat breakdown beyond our influence, but changes in diet and exercise decide each gasoline's overall usage. Surely, both of these considerations will be discussed more extensively below.

1. Quantity of nutrients consumed

Humans will obtain four calories from sources in their surroundings: carbon, hydrogen, nitrogen, and oxygen. When it comes to the body demanding and using a given energy supply, it prefers to choose the nearest one to it due to the quantity and concentration in the bloodstream. The body can improve its use of glucose or decrease its use of glucose directly due to the amount of carbohydrate intake being ingested. It is an effort by the liver to control glycogen (sugar) levels in the body. If carbohydrate (carb) intake goes up, the use of carbohydrate-containing goods will go up, in exchange. Proteins are slightly harder to control. As protein consumption goes up, our bodies increase their development and oxidation of proteins as well. The food source for our body is protein. If it is in short supply, our body will consume less of it. This is an attempt to keep body protein cellular levels stable at 24-hour intervals. Since dietary fat does not lift the amount of fat the body needs, it cannot dramatically change how much fuel the body gets from that fat. Rather than measuring insulin directly, it is important to measure insulin indirectly, so it does not drift.

The blood alcohol content can decrease the body's energy reserves with those calories of fat. This will almost entirely impair the body's usage of fat for food. As most people know, carbohydrate intake will influence the amount of fat the body uses as a fuel supply. High carb diets increase the body's use of fat for food and the insulin threshold and amount. Therefore, the highest fat oxidation rates occur when there are low levels of carbohydrates in the body. Another clarification of this can be found in chapter 18, where it is clarified that the amount of glycogen regulates how much fat is used by the muscles. When a human eats less energy and carbohydrates, the body can subsequently take up fat calories for food instead of carbohydrates.

2. Hormone levels

Factors like food, exercise, medications and hormones all play a part in how we use our bodies' fuel. The hormone known as insulin is of high interest to many physicians because it plays a significant role in a wide range of activities, including the bodies functioning. A glance at the hormones involved in fuel consumption is included in the following passage.

Insulin is a peptide (as in the "peptide" in "peptides" that are essential in digestion) that the pancreas releases in response to changes in blood glucose. As blood glucose goes up, insulin levels also rise, and the body will use this extra glucose to kind of store it as glycogen in the muscles or in the liver. Glucose and extra glucose will be forced into fat cells for preservation (as alpha-glycerophosphate). Protein synthesis is enhanced, and as a result, amino acids (the building blocks of proteins) are transferred out of the blood via muscle cells and are then placed together to make bigger proteins. Fat synthesis or "lipogenesis" (making fat) and fat accumulation are also induced. In effect, it's hard for insulin to be released from fat cells due to even tiny levels of it. The main objective of insulin is regulating blood glucose in a very small range of around 80 to 120 milligrams per decilitre. When blood glucose levels rise outside of the normal range, insulin is released to get the glucose levels back into a normal range. The greatest rise in blood glucose levels (and the greatest increase in insulin) happens when humans eat carbohydrates in the diet. Due to amino acids that can be converted to glycogen, the breakdown of proteins can cause an increase the amount of insulin released. FFA can induce insulin release and produce ketone bodies found at concentrations that are far smaller than those produced by carbohydrates or proteins.

When your glucose level decreases, as it does with exercise and from eating less carbohydrate, your insulin levels decrease as well. During cycles with low insulin and higher hormones, the body's storage fuels can burst, leading to a breakdown of stored fuels. After accumulation within the body, triglycerides are broken down into fatty acids and glycerol and released into the bloodstream. Specific proteins might be broken down into individual amino acids and used as sources of sources glucose. Glycogen is a material contained in the liver that is broken when insulin is absent. Failure to produce insulin suggests a pathological state. Type me, diabetes (or Insulin Dependent Diabetes Mellitus, IDDM). In a group of patients with Type I diabetes (1), these patients have a deficiency in the pancreas, causing them to be entire without insulin. I already told you that to practical control glucose levels, people with diabetes have to inject themselves with insulin. This is relevant in the next chapter since the difference between diabetic ketoacidosis and dietary mediated ketosis is made in the chapter after this. Glucagon is essentially known as insulin's mirror hormone in the body and has nearly opposite effects. The enzyme insulin is also a peptide hormone made by the pancreas, which is released from the cells of the body, and its primary function as well is to sustain stable glucose levels. However, once blood glucose goes down below average, glucagon increases blood glucose on its own. The precursors are expelled from the cells into the bloodstream.

Glucagon's key function is in the liver, where it signals the degradation of liver glycogen and the resulting release into the bloodstream. The release of glucagon is modulated by what we eat, the sort of workout, and the presence of a meal that activates the development of glucagon in the body (24). High amounts of insulin suppress the pancreas from releasing the hormone glucagon. Normally, glucagon's actions are restricted to the liver; by comparison, its function in these other tissues is yet to be detected (i.e., fat and muscle cells). On the other hand, when insulin levels are very low, such as when glucose restriction and activity occur, glucagon plays a minor role in fat mobilization, as well as the degradation of muscle glycogen. Glucagon's primary function is to regulate blood glucose under conditions of low blood sugar. But it also plays a crucial role in ketone body development in the liver, which we will address in-depth in the next chapter. Below are the definitions of two contrasting hormones. It should be obvious from reading the sentences that they have opposite effects on one another. Whereas insulin is a key storage hormone that allows for the retention of accumulated glucose, potassium, albumin and fat in the body, glucagon serves the same role by allowing for the utilization of stored fat in an organism.

Insulin and glucagon are central to the determination to be anabolic or catabolic. However, their presence in the body is not alone enough for muscle development. Other hormones are involved as well. They will briefly be discussed below. Growth hormone, which is a peptide hormone, elicits various effects on the body, such as its effects on blood flow and muscle tissue growth. The hormone to hold appetite at bay, Ghrelin, is released in response to several stressors. Most notably, exercise, a reduction in blood glucose, and carbohydrate restriction or fasting can both induce Ghrelin production. As its name suggests (GH), GH is a growth-promoting hormone, which enhances protein production (protein synthesis) in the body and liver. Glucose, glycogen, and triglycerides also are mobilized from fat cells for nutrition.

Adrenaline and noradrenaline (also called epinephrine and norepinephrine) are members of a special family of hormones called 'fight or flight' hormones. They tend to be released in response to discomfort, such as running, fasting, or consuming cold foods. Epinephrine is a drug that is emitted from the adrenal medulla, passing across the bloodstream to the brain to exert its effects on several tissues of the body. The impacts of the catecholamine's on the different tissues of the body are very involved and maybe the subject of a research paper. The primary function of catecholamine metabolites affecting the ketogenic diet was to increase fatty acids excretion in the urine and increase fatty acids in the blood. When it's hard for someone to change their ways, it's because their insulin levels aren't where they should be. The only hormone that actually affects fat mobilization is insulin. Like the Catecholamine's, insulin and insulin mimics have a corresponding effect on fat mobilization.

3. Liver glycogen

The liver is one of the most metabolically active organs in the whole human body. Although everything we consume is not digested immediately by the stomach, this is part of the whole digestion process. Like the body, the degree to which the liver retains glycogen is the dominating influence to the extent to which the body will retain or break down nutrients. It is typically (hesitation) because there is a higher body fat level associated with elevated liver glycogen levels. The liver is analogous to a short term stead storehouse and glycogen source regulating blood glucose in our body. After the liver releases more glucose into the blood, more glucagon is released, which activates the breaking down of liver glycogen to glucose, to be introduced into the bloodstream. When the liver has glycogen stocks completely, blood glucose levels are retained, and the body enters the anabolic state, meaning the incoming glucose, amino acids, and free fatty acids are all processed as these three molecules, respectively. This is often referred to as 'the fed establishment.' Red blood cells can't hold as much oxygen as they did when filled with massive amounts of glycogen, so they release it when they're no longer needed and transform into the liver. The body cuts edible protein into amino acids, which are then placed into the formation of amino acids, and finally, will produce for you fats and sugars. This is often referred to as the 'fasted' condition.

4. Enzyme levels

Precise control of fuel consumption in the body is done through the action of enzymes. Ultimately, enzyme levels are calculated by the carbohydrates that are being consumed in the diet and the hormone levels which are caused by it. On the other hand, where there is a surplus of carbohydrates in one's diet, this form of dietary shift stimulates insulin's influence on the cells' ability to utilize glucose and prevent fatty stores' degradation. Thus, if there is a decrease in insulin levels, the enzymes are blocked, which results in a drop in the enzymes involved in glucose usage and in fats breakdown. A long term adjustment to a high carbohydrate / low carbohydrate diet may induce longer-term modifications in the enzymes involved in fats and carbohydrates, resulting in long term changes in the core. If you limit carbohydrate consumption for many weeks, this will deplete enzymes' liver and muscle and transfer them to be brought upon the liver and muscle that concerns fat burning. The result of disrupting the balance of dietary components is an inability to use carbs for fuel for some time after food is reintroduced to the diet.

Chapter 3: Keto with Intermittent Fasting

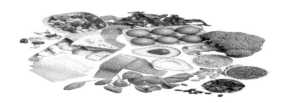

This chapter will give you a detailed view to the Keto with intermittent fasting.

Intermittent fasting, in a more condensed definition, allows people to miss a meal daily. The popular forms of intermittent fasting include the one day fast, a 24 hour fast or a 5:2 fast, where people eat very little food for a predetermined number of days, then consume lots of food (ADF). The intermittent fasting function of IF breaks the subjects fasting routine every other day. Unlike crash diets that frequently produce rapid results but can be hard to sustain for the long run, both intermittent fasting and keto Diet focus on the real root systems of how the body absorbs food and how you make your dietary decisions for each day. Intermittent eating and Keto diets should be practiced as dietary modification. They are long-term options for a better, happier you.

It is where the biggest distinction lies among IF and Interval feeding (TRF). The TRF is the fast of restricting the feeding time to between 4-10 hours during the day and missing the fasting time the rest of the time. All or most people who observe intermittent fasting do so regularly.

3.1. What Is Ketosis?

From the outside looking in, carbs appear to be a simple and fast means of bringing nutrients right through the day. Think of all those grab-and-go and protein-filled snacks that we equate with breakfast—granola bars, fruit-filled muffins, smoothies. We start our mornings by eating many carbs, and then later on in the day, they add more carbs. Just because a given technology works does not make it the most effective way. To keep us safe, the tissues and cells that produce our bodies require energy to fulfil their daily functions. There are two main sources of strength in the foods we consume, but the first source is non-animal, and the second source is animal. One source of energy is the carbohydrate, which transforms into glucose. At this time, this is the process that most people go through. These cars have an alternative fuel, however, and a shocking one: fat. No, the very thing any doctor has recommended you to reduce your lifelong lifespan may be the weapon you need to jump-start your metabolism. During this process, tiny organic molecules, called Ketone, are emitted from our body, signalling that the food we eat is being broken down. Ketones are actual nutrients that help run much of our body's cells, including muscles. You've undoubtedly heard the term "Metabolism" repeated in one's life, but do you understand what it means exactly as a fast-acting chemical process? In short, this is alkaline, causing effective cellular functioning, which can be present in any type of living thing. Considering that humans are extremely difficult in many ways, our bodies generally process simpler things like food and exercise. Our bodies are actively struggling to do their jobs. And whether we are either asleep or not, our cells are actively constructing and restoring. The robots ought to remove the energetic particles from inside our bodies.

Around the same time, glucose, which is what carbohydrates are broken down into after we ingest them, is a critical component in the process of bringing sugar into the body. We are now concentrating our diet on carbs as the main source of calories for our body. Without mentioning the fructose we eat as well as the recommended daily servings of fruit, starchy veggies, and starchy vegetables, as well as plant-based sources of protein, there is no shortage of glucose in our bodies. The problem with this type of energy use is that this results in us buying into the recycling-focused consumerism that is a by-product of the half-baked technologies. Our bodies get hammered by the number of calories we eat every day. Some people are eating more than they need, and that can contribute to obesity.

Most people cannot reach ketosis quickly, but you can reach it by exercising, eating less, and drinking a decent amount of water. As was seen through the data, our current "Food Pyramid," which instructs us to consume a high amount of carbohydrate-rich foods as energy sources, is turned upside down. A more effective formula for feeding your body has fats at the top, making up 60 to 80 percent of your diet; protein in the middle at 20 to 30 percent; and carbs (real glucose in disguise) way at the bottom, accounting for only 5 to 10 percent of your regular eating plan.

3.2. Paleo vs. Keto

Evolution has many opportunities to bring. We can use fire and energy to cook our food is evidence enough that change can be a positive thing about our lives. Anywhere between our trapper foraging lifestyle and the industrialized lifestyle we have today, there is a significant disconnect. Although our lifespans have improved, we're not winning from the longevity of those additional years because our health is being undermined. The tired, unclear sensation you are having might be not just because you need to get more sleep - it may be because you lack vitamin B12 in your diet. If we eat food as fuel for our bodies, it's fair to assume that what we eat has a big effect on our productivity. If you burn fuel in an engine designed to run on gasoline, there could be some very harmful consequences. Is it conceivable that our bodies have set up this insulin receptor cascade to only accept sugar, in a process comparable to our transition to providing fat as a rapid source of energy rather than a source of energy for our early ancestors? I know this sounds an awful lot like arguing for a Paleo diet, but although the ketogenic lifestyle seems similar, keto's basic concept is vastly different. Ketosis happens when you eat fewer calories and change the intake of protein and fat. There are many medicinal effects of ketosis, and the primary one is quick weight loss (fat, protein, carbohydrates, fiber, and fluids). Per calorie is made up of four distinct types of macronutrients. Many considerations go into the certain food decisions that a person makes, and it's crucial to consider one's emotions.

Fiber makes us regular, for instance, and it lets food flows into the digestive tract. What goes in has to come out, and for that process, fiber is necessary. Protein helps to heal tissue, generate enzymes and to create bones, muscles and skin. Liquids keep us hydrated; our cells, muscles, and organs do not operate correctly without them. The primary function of carbohydrates is to supply energy, but the body must turn them into glucose to do so, which has a ripple effect on the body's parts. Because of its link to insulin production through higher blood sugar levels, a carb intake is a balancing act for persons with diabetes. Good fats stimulate cell formation, protect our lungs, help keep us warm, and supply nutrition, but only in small amounts when carbs are ingested. I'm going to explain more about when and how this is happening soon.

3.3. Carbs vs. Net Carbs

In virtually any food supply, carbohydrates occur in some type. Total carbohydrate reduction is unlikely and unrealistic. To work, we want some carbohydrates. If we want to learn that certain foods that drop into the restricted group on a keto diet become better options than others, it's important to understand this.

In the caloric breakdown of a meal, fiber counts as a carb. It is interesting to remember is that our blood sugar is not greatly impaired by fiber, a positive thing because it is an integral macronutrient that allows us better digest food. You're left with what's considered net carbs after subtracting the sum of fiber from the number of carbs in the caloric tally of an element or finished recipe. Think of your pay check before (gross) taxes and after (net). A bad comparison, maybe, because no one wants to pay taxes, but an efficient one to try to explain and track carbs versus net carbs. You place a certain amount of carbohydrates in your bloodstream, but any of them does not influence your blood sugar content.

It doesn't mean that with whole-grain pasta, you may go mad. Although it's a better alternative than flour of white-coloured pasta, you can limit your net carbs to 20 - 30 grams per day total. To place that in context, approximately 35 g of carbohydrates and just 7 grams of total fiber are found in two ounces of undercooked whole-grain pasta. Pasta and bread are undoubtedly the two key things people would ask you if you miss them.

3.4. When does ketosis kick in?

Most individuals go through ketosis within a few days. People who are different will take a week to adapt. Factors that cause ketosis include existing body mass, diet, and exercise levels. Ketosis is a moderate state of ketosis since ketone levels would be low for a longer time. One can calculate ketone levels in a structured way, but you can note certain biological reactions that indicate you are in ketosis. There are not as serious or drastic symptoms, and benefits can outweigh risks in this phase-in time, so it is good to be familiar with symptoms in case they arise.

Starvation vs. Fasting

Make a deliberate decision to fast. The biggest differentiator between going on a fast and feeding intermittently is that it is your choice to continue fasting. The amount of time you want to fast and the reason for fasting are not imposed upon you by the hospital, whether it is for religious practices, weight loss, or a prolonged detox cycle. Most fasting is performed at will. When fasting, proper feeding has clear implications on the overall way of our well-being. A series of situations can bring about starvation out of the hands of the people suffering from those conditions. Starvation, hunger, and war are but a couple of these conditions to be caused by a devastated economy. Starvation is starvation due to lack of the proper nutrients that can lead to organ failure and ultimately death. No one wants to live without calories.

When I knew that avoiding smoking would help my health, I immediately wondered, "Why do I continue to smoke?"

And once I learn about the motivations for doing this, it is much easier to see them. I have also been concerned about the early days of fasting. Before I knew that there is a distinction between fasting and starvation and that it is safe, my first response to the thought of not eating and starving was still, "Why would anyone choose to kill themselves with starving?." As for this article's intent, someone who fasts is just opting not to eat for a predetermined amount of time. Even nonviolent vigils that are meant to oppose using a certain form of killing feed larger and larger gatherings.

Would your hunger vanish before the fast?

So that's a brilliant query; let's try a couple more angles. The fact is, we all eat a full meal once a day. It is a normal tradition that we eat our last meal a few hours before going to sleep, and all but breastfeeding new-borns do not eat the moment they wake up. And if you devote just a limit of six hours a night to sleep, you are likely to be fasting ten hours a day anyway. Now, let's begin to incorporate the concept in periodic to the formula. Anything that is "intermittent" implies something that is not constant. When adding it to the concept of fasting, it means you're lengthening the time that you don't eat between meals (the term "breakfast" means only that, breaking the fast).

From fasting once a day, we have an established "mind over matter" power. What will be a major concern, though, would be mind over mind. We will come back to the issue of how you feel after you stop feeding. The first week of fasting may change as you get used to the prolonged amount of time of your current intermittent fasting target. All of the fasting periods that I have given allow you timewise to adapt to the Ketogenic Diet and this method adjusts your sleeping routine so that it suits them. It is conceivable (and likely) that your body will start to feel hungry about 10 a.m., around the moment it usually eats lunch. But, after one day, you can adapt, and after a couple of days, you should no longer have trouble feeding before noon.

To support you before making the shift you're playing with, observe what happens when you put back the first meal of the day by an extra thirty minutes per day for a week. This way, as you begin the schedule set out here, you'll need to change the timing of your final meal of the day just after you begin week two of the plan for the Meals from Noon to 6 p.m. No appointments are required.

3.5. Why Prefer Intermittent Fasting?

Now that you have learned that it is possible to fast without starving to death and that it is also a deliberate decision, you might think, why on earth you would ever choose to fast. Its ability to encourage weight loss is one of the key reasons that IF has taken the diet world by storm. Metabolism is one feature of the human body. Metabolism requires two basic reactions: catabolism and anabolism.

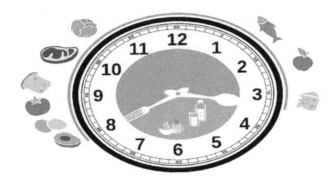

Catabolism is the portion of metabolism where our bodies break down food. Catabolism involves breaking down large compounds into smaller units. The body uses the energy from the food we consume to produce new cells, build muscles, and sustain organs. This term is often referred to as parallel or dual catabolism and anabolism. A diet routine that sees us eating most of the day means our bodies have less time to waste in the anabolic process of metabolism. It is hard to find out since they are related, but note that they occur at different rates. The most significant point is that a prolonged fasting time allows for optimum metabolic efficiency.

The improved mental acuity has an intrinsic influence of improving attention, focus, concentration and focus. According to various reports, fasting made you more alert and concentrated, not sleepy or light-headed. Many people point to nature and our desire to survive. We may not have had food preservation, but we lived day to day, regardless of how ample food supplies may have been.

Scientists agree that fasting often heightens neurogenesis, the growth and regeneration of nerve tissue in the brain. Both paths lead to the fact that fasting gives the body enough time to do routine maintenance. You extend the time you give your body to concentrate on cellular growth and tissue recovery by sleeping longer between your last meal and your first meal.

Are Fluids Allowed While Fasting?

The last important detail for intermittent fasting is that it speeds up the metabolism; unlike religious fasting, which also forbids food consumption during the fast period, an IF requires you to drink a certain liquid during the fast time. You are not consuming something that is caloric; therefore, this action breaks the fast. As we can glean from its strong weight loss record, a closer look through the prism of intermittent fasting can yield very promising outcomes. Bone broth (here) is the beneficiary of both the nutrients and vitamins and can refill the sodium amounts. Permission has been given to use coffee and tea without any sweeteners and ideally without any milk or cream. There are two separate schools of thinking about applying milk or soda to your coffee or tea. Provided it's just a high-fat addition, such as coconut oil or butter to make bulletproof coffee (here), many keto supporters believe it's a waste of time and not properly gain sufficient protein. Using MCT oil, it is assumed that people can obtain more energy and be happier moving on with their daily lives. Coffee and tea drinkers tend toward simple brews. It is perfect for you to choose whichever strategy you want, as long as you don't end up "alternating" between the two techniques. I often recommend drinking water, as staying hydrated is necessary for any healthier choice a person can make. Caffeine use can be very depleting, so be careful to control your water intake and keep yourself balanced.

3.6. The Power of Keto Combined & Intermittent Fasting

When you're in ketosis, the process breaks down fatty acids to create ketones for fuel is basically what the body does to keep things going when you're fasting. Fasting for a few days has a noticeable impact on a carb-based diet. After the initial step of burning carbohydrates for energy, your body transforms to burning fat for heat. You see where I'm going. If it takes 24 to 48 hrs. For the body to turn to fat for food, imagine the consequences of keto. Maintaining ketosis means your body has been trying to burn fat for fuel. Spending a long time in a fasting state means you burn fat. Intermittent starvation combined with keto results in more weight loss than other traditional diets. Extra fat-burning capabilities are due to the gap in time between the last and first meals. Ketosis is used in bodybuilding because it helps shed fat without losing muscle. It's healthy when it's the right weight, and muscle mass is good for fitness.

How does it work?

It is an incredible lifestyle adjustment to turn to the keto diet. Since it can help you consume less, it's better to ease into this program's fasting part. Despite the diet not being entirely fresh, yet has been around for a long time, people seem to respond rapidly to consuming mostly fat, so their body has been accustomed to burning fat for food, but be patient if either of the above occurs: headaches, exhaustion, light-headedness, dizziness, low blood sugars, nausea. A rise in appetite, cravings for carbohydrates, or weight gain. Often make sure you get certain nutrients: brain well-being, fat-burning, testosterone, and mood. Week 2 of the 4-Week schedule begins intermittent fasting, and it is not continued until the 2nd week. During the phase-in process, you'll want to find out what the meals and hours are about. Before integrating the intermittent-fasting portion of your diet, it is recommended that you stop eating your last meal more than six hours in advance. (6 p.m.) It will help you get into a fasting state and help you stop snacking. When you learn how to better nourish your body, you will learn how to reel in the pesky compulsion to feed, and you will be able to maintain a more controlled relationship with your psychological needs as well. When time goes by, cravings inevitably stop. We sometimes associate the craving for food with hunger, when actually the craving for food is due to a learned habit and hunger is a biochemical cue to refuel the body's energy stores.

3.7. Calories vs. Macronutrients

The focus on keto is on tracking the amount of fat, protein, and carbohydrates you eat. It's just a closer examination of every calorie ingested. To decide how many calories you can consume for weight management and weight loss, it is also important to have a baseline metabolic rate called BMR (another reason defining your goals is important). In both your general well-being and achieving and remaining in ketosis, all these macronutrients play a crucial function, but carbohydrates are the one that receives the most attention on keto since they result in glucose during digestion, which is the energy source you are attempting to guide your body away from utilizing. Any study indicates that the actual number of total carbs that one can eat a day on keto is 50 grams or less, resulting in 20 to 35 net carbs a day depending on the fiber content. The lower the net carbohydrates you can get down, the sooner your body goes into ketosis, and the better it's going to be to keep in it.

Bearing in mind that we target around 20 grams of net carbs a day, depending on how many calories you need to eat depending on your BMR, the fat and protein grams are factors. Depending on the exercise level, the recommended daily average for women ranges between 1,600 and 2,000 calories for weight maintenance (from passive to active). According to a daily diet, consuming 160 grams of fat + 70 grams of protein + 20 grams of carbohydrates represents 1,800 calories of intake, the optimal number for weight control for moderately active women in the USDA (walking 1.5 to 3 miles a day). You would like to reach for 130 grams of fat + 60 grams of protein + 20 grams of carbohydrates to jump-start weight loss if you have a sedentary lifestyle, described as having exercise from normal daily activities such as cleaning and walking short distances only (1500 calories).

3.8. The Physical Side Effects of Keto:

Unlike diet programs that merely reduce the weight loss foods you consume, keto goes further. In order to improve how the body turns what you consume into electricity, ketosis is about modifying the way you eat. The ketosis phase changes the equation from burning glucose (remember, carbs) to burning fat for fuel instead. When the body adapts to a different way of working, this comes with potential side effects. This is also why around week two, and not from the get-go, the 4-Week schedule here stages of intermittent fasting. It's important to give yourself time to change properly, both physically and mentally. Keto fever and keto breath are two physical alterations that you may encounter while transitioning to a keto diet.

1. Keto Flu

Often referred to as carb flu, keto flu can last anywhere from a few days to a few weeks. As the body weans itself from burning glucose for energy, metabolic changes occurring inside can result in increased feelings of lethargy, muscle soreness, irritability, light-headedness or brain fog, changes in bowel movements, nausea, stomach aches, and difficulty concentrating and focusing. It sounds bad, I know, and perhaps slightly familiar. Yes, these are all recurrent flu signs, hence the term. The good news is that when your body changes, this is a transient process, and it does not affect everybody. A deficiency of electrolytes (sodium, potassium, magnesium and calcium) and sugar removal from substantially reduced carbohydrate intake are reasons causing these symptoms. Expecting these future effects means that, should anything arise at all, you

183

will be prepared to relieve them and reduce the duration of keto flu.

Sodium levels are specifically affected by the volume of heavily processed foods you eat. To explain, all we eat is a processed food; the word means "a series of steps taken to achieve a specific end." The act of processing food also involves cooking from scratch at home. However, these heavily processed foods appear to produce excessive amounts of secret salt in contrast to our present society, where ready-to-eat foods are available at any turn of the store (sodium is a preservative as well as a flavour modifier).

Other foods to concentrate on during your keto phase-in time are given below. They're a rich supply of minerals such as magnesium, potassium and calcium to keep the electrolytes in check.

- Potassium is important for hydration. It is present in Brussels sprouts, asparagus, salmon, tomatoes, avocados, and leafy greens.
- Seafood, Avocado, Spinach, Fish, and Vegetables that are high in magnesium can greatly assist with Cramps and Muscle Soreness.
- Calcium can promote bone health and aid in the absorption of nutrients.
- Including cheese, nuts, and seeds like almonds, broccoli, bok Choy, sardines, lettuce, sesame and chia seeds.

The other option that people evaluate to prevent the keto flu is to start eating less refined carbohydrates to lessen the chances of experiencing the keto flu. It can be as simple as making a few simple changes in what you eat, replacing the muffin with a hard-boiled or scrambled egg, replacing the bun with lettuce (often referred to as protein-style when ordering), or switching out spaghetti with zoodles. This way, when you dive into the plan here or here, it'll feel more like a gradual step of eating fewer carbohydrates than a sudden right turn in your diet.

2. Keto Breath

Let's dig into the crux of the matter first. Poor breath is basically a stench. But, it's a thing you can prepare yourself for when transitioning to the ketosis diet. There are two related hypotheses there might be a reason for this. When the body reaches ketosis (a state whereby it releases a lot of energy), which makes your fat a by-product of acid, more acetone is released by the body (yes, the same solvent found in nail polish remover and paint thinners). Any acetone is broken down in the bloodstream in a process called decarboxylation in order to get it out of the body into the urine and breathe in the acetone. It can cause that a person has foul-smelling breath.

When protein is also present in the keto breath, it adds a mildly gross sound. You must note that the macronutrient target is a high fat, mild protein, and low carb. People make the mistake that high fat is interchangeable with high protein. It is not a real assertion at all. The body's metabolism between fat and protein varies. Our bodies contain ammonia when breaking down protein, and all of the ammonia is normally released in our urine production. When you eat more protein or more than you should, the excess protein is not broken or digested and goes to your gut. With time, the extra protein will turn to ammonia and releasing by your breath.

3.9. The Fundamentals of Ketogenic Diet

The keto diet regimen involves eating moderately low carb, high sugar, and mild protein to train the body to accept fat as its basic food. Continuing the procedure, I would add a

Keto diet to my diet. Since the body may not have carbohydrate stores, it burns through its glycogen supplies rapidly. It is when the body appears to be in a state of emergency since it has run out of food. At this stage, the body goes into ketosis, and this is when you start using fat as the primary source of power. It typically occurs within three days of beginning the drug. Then, the body transforms the fat onto itself, usually taking over three months and a half to complete the transition. You are well accustomed to fat. So if you aren't feeding the body properly, that's why the body takes advantage of your own fat deposits (fasting).

The Keto Diet Advantage for Intermittent Fasting

Before entering intermittent fasting, keto advises four a month and a half to be on the keto diet. You're not going to be better off eating fat alone, so you're going to have less yearning. The keto diet in contemplates was all the more satisfying, and people encountered less yearning. In contrast, keto also showed its bulk storage ability and was best at maintaining digestion.

Sorts of Intermittent Fasting

This technique involves fasting two days a week and on some days actually eating 500 calories. You will have to observe a typical, healthy keto diet for the next five days. Because fasting days are allotted just 500 calories, you will need to spend high-protein and fat nutrients to keep you satisfied. Only made mindful that there is a non-fasting day in the middle of both.

1. Time-Restricted Eating

For the most part, because your fasting window involves the time you are dozing, this fasting approach has proven to be among the most popular. The swift 16/8 means that you are fast for sixteen hours and eat for eight hours. That might believe it is only allowed to eat from early afternoon until 8 p.m. and start quickly until the next day. The incredible thing about this technique is that it doesn't have to be 16/8; at the moment, you can do 14/10 and get equivalent incentives.

2. Interchange Day Fasting

Despite the 5:2 strategy and time restriction, this alternative allows you to be rapid every other day, normally limiting yourself from around 500 calories on fasting. The non-fasting days would actually be consumed normally. It can be an exhausting strategy that can make others hesitate when it is difficult to keep up with it.

3. 24 Hour Fast

I called, for short, "One Meal a Day" or OMAD, otherwise. This speed is sustained for an entire 24 hours and is usually done just a few days a week. Next, you'll need some inspiration to resume fasting to prop you up.

Keeping up the Motivation

It can be hard to stick to an eating and fasting regimen on the off chance that you are short on ideas, so how do you keep it up? The accompanying focus will help to concentrate on your general goals by presenting basic path reasons.

Chapter 4: Top 20 Keto Recipes

In this chapter, we will discuss some delicious keto recipes.

4.1. Muffins of Almond Butter

(Ready in 35 Mins, Serves: 12, Difficulty: Normal)

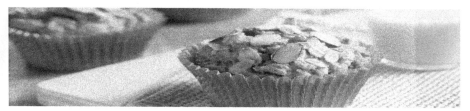

Ingredients:

- Four eggs
- 2 cups almond flour
- 1/4 tsp. salt
- 3/4 cup warm almond butter,
- 3/4 cup almond milk
- 1 cup powdered erythritol
- Two teaspoons baking powder

Instructions:

1. In a muffin cup, put the paper liners before the oven is preheated to 160 degrees Celsius.

2. Mix erythritol, almond meal, baking powder, and salt in a mixing bowl.

3. In another cup, mix the warm almond milk with the almond butter.

4. Drop some ingredients in a dry bowl till they are all combined.

5. In a ready cooker, sprinkle the flour and cook for 22-25 minutes until a clean knife is placed in the center.

6. Cool the bottle for five minutes to cool.

4.2. Breakfast Quesadilla

(Ready in 25 Mins, Serves: 4, Difficulty: Easy)

Ingredients:

- 4 eggs
- 1/4 cup (56 g) salsa
- 1/4 cup (30 g) low-fat Cheddar cheese, shredded
- 8 corn tortillas

Instructions:

1. When it is done, throw in the salsa, and whisk in the cheese to the very top. Sprinkle the oil on a few tortillas and then place a few pieces on an even number of the tortillas' edges.

2. Take the baking sheet. Divide the egg mixture between the tortillas, which is much more challenging. Oil-side up, cover the remaining tortillas. For 3 minutes or before the golden brown heats up, grill the quesadillas on each side. Serve.

4.3. California Breakfast Sandwich

(Ready in 30 Mins, Serves: 6, Difficulty: Easy)

Ingredients:

- 1/2 a cup (90 g) chopped tomato
- 1/2 a cup (60 g) grated Cheddar cheese
- Six whole-wheat English muffins

- 2 ounces (55 g) mushrooms, sliced
- One avocado, sliced
- 6 eggs
- 3/4 cup (120 g) chopped onion
- 1 tbsp. unsalted butter

Instructions:

Beat the eggs together. Brown onion in a large oven-proof or high-sided skillet until clear. It's safe and tidy. Chop up avocado, tomatoes, and champagne onion blend and stir. Blend together. Proofread the attached work. Quickly cook until it's almost cooked. Add the salt, vinegar, and cheese. Spoon with English toasted muffins.

4.4. Stromboli Keto

(Ready in 45 Mins, Serves: 4, Difficulty: Normal)

Ingredients:

- 4 oz. ham
- 4 oz. cheddar cheese
- Salt and pepper
- 4 tbsp. almond flour
- 1¼ cup shredded mozzarella cheese
- 1 tsp. Italian seasoning
- 3 tbsp. coconut flour
- One egg

•

Instructions:

1. To avoid smoking, stir the mozzarella cheese in the microwave for 1 minute or so.

2. Apply each cup of the melted mozzarella cheese, mix the food, coconut fleece, pepper and salt together. A balanced equilibrium. Then add the eggs and blend again for a while after cooling off.

3. Place the mixture on the parchment pad and place the second layer above it. Through your hands or rolling pin, flatten it into a rectangle.

4. Remove the top sheet of paper and use a butter knife to draw diagonal lines towards the dough's middle. They can be cut one-half of the way on the one side. And cut diagonal points on the other side, too.

5. At the edge of the dough are alternate ham and cheese slices. Then fold on one side, and on the other side, cover the filling.

6. Bake for 15-20 minutes at 226°C; place it on a baking tray.

4.5. Cups of Meat-Lover Pizza

(Ready in 26 Mins, Serves: 12, Difficulty: Easy)

Ingredients:

- 24 pepperoni slices
- 1 cup cooked and crumbled bacon
- 12 tbsp. sugar-free pizza sauce
- 3 cups grated mozzarella cheese
- 12 deli ham slices

- 1 lb. bulk Italian sausage

Instructions

1. Preheat the oven to 375 F Celsius (190 degrees Celsius). Italian brown sausages, soaked in a saucepan of extra fat.

2. Cover the 12-cup ham slices with a muffin tin. Divide it into sausage cups, mozzarella cheese, pizza sauce, and pepperoni slots.

3. Bake for 10 mins at 375. Cook for 1 minute until the cheese pops and the meat tops show on the ends, until juicy.

4. Enjoy the muffin and put the pizza cups to avoid wetting them on paper towels. Uncover or cool down and heat up quickly in the toaster oven or microwave.

4.6. Chicken Keto Sandwich

(Ready in 30 Mins, Serves: 2, Difficulty: Normal)

Ingredients:

For the Bread:

- 3 oz. cream cheese
- ⅛ tsp. cream of tartar Salt
- Garlic powder
- Three eggs

For the Filling:

- 1 tbsp. mayonnaise
- Two slices bacon
- 3 oz. chicken
- 1 tsp. Sriracha
- 2 slices pepper jack cheese
- 2 grape tomatoes
- ¼ avocado

Instructions:

1. Divide the eggs into several cups. Add cream tartar, cinnamon, then beat to steep peaks in the egg whites.

2. In a different bowl, beat the cream cheese. In a white egg mixture, combine the mixture carefully.

3. Place the batter on paper and, like bread pieces, make little square shapes. Gloss over the garlic powder, then bake for 25 mins at 148°C.

4. As the bread bakes, cook the chicken and bacon in a saucepan and season to taste.

5. Remove from the oven and cool when the bread is finished for 10-15 mins. Then add mayo, Sriracha, tomatoes, and mashed avocado, and add fried chicken and bacon to your sandwich.

4.7. Keto Tuna Bites With Avocado

(Ready in 13 Mins, Serves: 8, Difficulty: Very Easy)

Ingredients:

- 10 oz. drained canned tuna
- ⅓ cup almond flour
- ½ cup coconut oil
- ¼ cup mayo
- 1 avocado
- ½ tsp. garlic powder
- ¼ tsp. onion powder
- ¼ cup parmesan cheese
- Salt and pepper

Instructions:

1. Both ingredients are mixed in a dish (excluding cocoa oil). Shape small balls of almond meal and fill them.

2. Fry them with coconut oil (it needs to be hot) in a medium-hot pan until browned on all sides.

4.8. Green Keto Salad

(Ready in 10 Mins, Serves: 1, Difficulty: Easy)

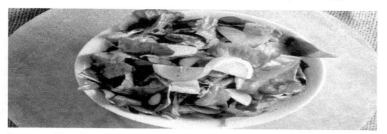

Ingredients:

- 100 g mixed lettuce
- 200 g cucumber
- 2 stalks celery
- 1 tbsp. olive oil
- Salt as per choice
- 1 tsp white wine vinegar or lemon juice

Instructions:

1. With your hands, rinse and cut the lettuce.

2. Cucumber and celery chop.

3. Combine all.

4. For the dressing, add vinegar, salt, and oil.

4.9. Breakfast Enchiladas

(Ready in 1 Hr., Serves: 8, Difficulty: Normal)

Ingredients:

- 12 ounces (340 g) ham, finely chopped
- Eight whole-wheat tortillas
- 4 eggs
- 1 tbsp. flour
- 1/4 tsp. garlic powder
- 1 tsp. Tabasco sauce
- 2 cups (300 g) chopped green bell pepper
- 1 cup (160 g) chopped onion
- 2 1/2 a cup (300 g) grated Cheddar cheese
- 2 cups (475 ml) skim milk
- 1/2 a cup (50 g) chopped scallions

Instructions:

1. Preheat the oven to 350 °F (180 °C). Combine the ham, scallions, bell pepper, tomatoes and cheese. Apply five teaspoons of the mixture to each tortilla and roll-up.

2. In a 30 x 18 x 5-cm (12 x 7 x 2-inch) non-stick pan. In a separate oven, beat together the eggs, milk, garlic, and Tabasco. Cook for 30 minutes with foil, then show the last 10 minutes.

Tip: Serve with a sour cream dollop, salsa, and slices of avocado.

4.10. Keto Mixed Berry Smoothie Recipe

(Ready in 5 Mins, Serves: 4, Difficulty: Easy)

Ingredients:

- 2 scoops Vanilla Collagen
- 1 cup of frozen Mixed Berries
- 2 cups Ice
- 1/4 cup Erythritol Powdered Monk Fruit
- 1 cup Unsweetened Coconut Milk Vanilla

Instructions

1. In a high-speed blender, combine all the ingredients.
2. Use or mix until smooth the "smoothie" setting.

4.11. Low-Carb Tropical Pink Smoothie

(Ready in 5 Mins, Serves: 1, Difficulty: Easy)

Ingredients: (makes 1 smoothie)

- $^1/_2$ small dragon fruit
- 1 tbsp. chia seeds
- 1 small wedge Gallia, Honeydew
- 1/2 a cup coconut milk *or* heavy whipping cream
- 1 scoop of whey protein powder (vanilla or plain), or gelatin or egg white powder.
- 3-6 drops extract of Stevia *or* other low-carb sweeteners
- 1/2 a cup water

- *Optional:* few ice cubes

Instructions

1. Monitor and place all the components smoothly in a mixer and pulse. Before or after combining this, you can apply the ice.

2. It is possible to include the fruit of a white or pink dragon. Serve.

4.12. Keto Peanut Butter Smoothie

(Ready in 1 Min, Serves: 1, Difficulty: Very Easy)

Ingredients:

- 1/2 a cup almond milk
- 1 tbsp. peanut butter
- 1 tbsp. cocoa powder
- 1-2 tbsp. peanut butter powdered
- 1/4 of avocado
- 1 serving liquid stevia
- 1/4 cup ice

Instructions

1. Add all the ingredients other than the ice and mix well in a food processor.

2. Apply enough milk to the smoothie for the ideal consistency. Add more ice or ground peanut butter to thin it out.

3. Serve it in a glass.

4.13. 5 Minute Keto Cookies & Cream Milkshake

(Ready in 5 Mins, Serves: 2, Difficulty: Easy)

Ingredients:

- $3/4$ cup heavy whipping cream or coconut milk
- Two large squares of grated dark chocolate
- **Optional:** frozen cubes of almond milk/ few ice cubes
- 1 cup unsweetened any nut or almond milk or seed milk
- 1 tsp vanilla powder or vanilla extract sugar-free
- 1-2 tsp Erythritol powdered, few drops of stevia
- $1/3$ cup walnuts or pecans chopped
- 2 tbsp. almond butter, (roasted or sunflower seed)
- 2 tbsp. coconut cream /whipped cream for garnishing

Instructions

1. Place in a blender, mix all the ingredients together (except topping). It is thicker as you blink. The ganache should be lit or topped with other ingredients.

2. Mix the whipped cream into the topping separately. Use 1/2 to 1 cup of milk for pounding. You should have whipped cream in the fridge for three days.

3. Pour some water into a bottle. Drizzle the nuts and butter leftover over the milk.

4.14. Keto Eggnog Smoothie

(Ready in 5 Mins, Serves: 1, Difficulty: Easy)

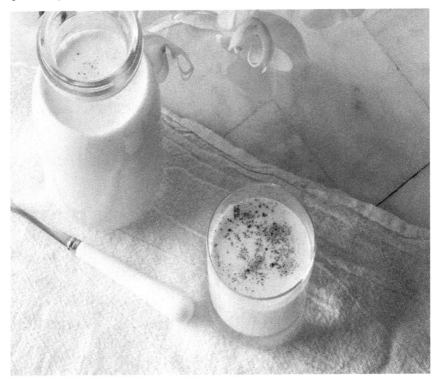

Ingredients:

- 1 Large Egg
- 1 tsp Erythritol
- 1/4 cup whipping cream (coconut cream for dairy-free)
- 1/2 tsp Cinnamon
- 4 Cloves ground approx. ¼ tsp
- 1 tsp Maple Syrup Sugar-Free (optional)

Instructions

In a blender, combine all the ingredients and mix fast for 30 seconds – 1 min.

4.15. Easy Keto Oreo Shake

(Ready in 5 Mins, Serves: 2, Difficulty: Easy)

Ingredients:

- 4 large eggs
- 2 tbsp. black cocoa powder or Dutch-process cocoa powder
- 1 1/2 cups unsweetened cashew milk, almond milk, or water 4 tbsp. roasted almond butter or Keto Butter
- 3 tbsp. Erythritol powdered or Swerve
- 1/4 cup whipping cream
- 1/4 tsp vanilla powder or 1/2 tsp vanilla extract (sugar-free)
- 1/2 a cup whipped cream for garnishing

●

Instructions

1. Place the frozen or cashew milk/almond milk in an ice cube tray and then freeze them. Under the right conditions (which means don't freeze the shake), miss this step and go on to the next.

2. Stir the cream in a tub of frozen milk. To produce ice cream, add ice cream to the warmed cream. Put some ova somewhere.

3. Apply the soaked nuts, sweetener, cacao powder, and vanilla to the dish. With macadamia, cocoa, cassava, and MCT, these oils are nice to use with MCT oil. Blend until smooth.

6. Apply more whipped cream before serving.

4.16. Keto Eggs Florentine

(Ready in 55 Mins, Serves: 4, Difficulty: Normal)

Ingredients:

- 1 tbsp. of white vinegar
- 1 Cup cleaned, the spinach leaves fresh
- 2 Tablespoons of Parmesan cheese, finely grated
- 2 Chickens
- 2 Eggs
- Ocean salt and chili to compare

Instructions:

1. Boil the spinach in a decent bowl or steam until it waves.

2. Sprinkle with the parmesan cheese to taste.

3. Break and put the bits on a tray. Place the tray on them.

4. Steam a hot water bath, add the vinegar and mix it in a whirlpool with a wooden spoon.

5. Place the egg in the center of the egg, turn the heat over and cover until set (3-4 minutes). Repeat for the second seed.

6. Put the spinach with the egg and drink.

4.17. Loaded Cauliflower (Low Carb, Keto)

(Ready in 20 Mins, Serves: 4, Difficulty: Easy)

Ingredients:

- 1 pound cauliflower

- 3 tablespoons butter
- 4 ounces of sour cream
- 1/4 tsp. garlic powder
- 1 cup cheddar cheese, grated
- 2 slices bacon crumbled and cooked
- 2 tbsp. chives snipped
- pepper and salt to taste

Instructions

1. Chop or dice cauliflower and switch to a microwave-safe oven. Add two water teaspoons and cover with sticking film. Microwave for 5-10 minutes until thoroughly cooked and tender. Empty the excess water, give a minute or two to dry. If you want to strain the cooking water, steam up your cooling flora (or use hot water as normal.)

2. Add the cauliflower to the food processor. Pulse it until smooth and creamy. Mix in the sugar, garlic powder and sour cream. Press it in a cup, then scatter with more cheese, then mix it up. Add pepper and salt.

3. Add the leftover cheese, chives and bacon to the loaded cauliflower. Place the cauliflower under the grill for a few minutes in the microwave to melt the cheese.

4. Serve and enjoy.

4.18. Crispy Drumsticks

(Ready in 1 Hr. 5 Mins, Serves: 4, Difficulty: Normal)

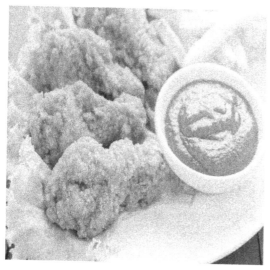

Ingredients:

- Dried thyme
- Olive oil
- 10 – 12 chicken drumsticks (preferably organic)
- Paprika
- Sea salt
- Black pepper
- 4 tbsp. Grass-fed butter or ghee, melted and divided

Instructions

1. Heat the oven to 375 F.

2. Line a rimmed baking sheet.

3. On the parchment paper, in a single sheet of holes between the drumsticks.

4. Mix 1/2 of the melted butter or ghee in olive oil with drumsticks.

5. Sprinkle on thyme and seasoning.

6. Turn it on for 30 minutes. Carefully empty the bottle and switch drumsticks over. When the drumsticks are cooling, produce a thyme and butter mixture again.

7. Return the pie for another 30 minutes (or until finely browned and externally baked).

4.18. Shredded Herbal Cattle

(Ready in 50 Mins, Serves: 4, Difficulty: Normal)

Ingredients:

- 2 tablespoons of rice wine
- 1 tbsp. of olive oil
- 1 pound leg,
- 2 Chipotle peppers in adobo sauce,
- 1 garlic clove chopped,
- Mature tomatoes, peeled and pureed
- 1 yellow onion
- 1/2 tbsp. chopped fresh Mustard
- 1 cup of dried basil
- 1 cup of dried marjoram
- 1/4 cut into strips beef
- 2 medium shaped chipotles crushed

- 1 cup beef bone broth
- Table salt and ground black pepper,
- Parsley, 2 spoonful's of new chives, finely chopped

Instructions:

In an oven, steam the oil in a medium to high heat. Continuously cook beef for six to seven minutes. Add all the ingredients to the beef. Heat and cook for 40 minutes; add the remaining to a moderate-low heat. Then tear the meat, have it.

4.19. Nilaga Filipino Soup

(Ready in 45 Mins, Serves: 4, Difficulty: Normal)

Ingredients:

- 1 Tsp. butter
- 1 tbsp. patis (fish sauce)
- 1 pound of pork ribs, boneless and 1 shallot thinly sliced bits,
- Split 2 garlic cloves, chopped 1 (1/2) "slice of fresh ginger, 1 cup chopped
- 1 cup of fresh tomatoes,
- 1 cup pureed "Corn."
- Cauliflower
- salt and green chili pepper, to taste

Instructions:

1. Melt the butter in a bowl over medium to high heat. Heat the pork ribs for 5-6 minutes on both sides. Stir in the shallot, the garlic and the ginger. Add extra ingredients.

2. Cook, sealed, for 30 to 35 mins. Serve in different containers and remain together.

4.20. Lemon Mahi-Mahi Garlicky

(Ready in 30 Mins, Serves: 4, Difficulty: Normal)

Ingredients:

- Kosher salt
- 4 (4-oz.) mahi-mahi fillets
- Ground black pepper
- 1 lb. asparagus
- 2 tbsp. extra-virgin olive oil,
- 1 lemon
- juice of 1 lemon and zest also
- 3 cloves garlic
- ¼ tsp. of crushed red pepper flakes
- 3 tbsp. butter, divided
- 1 tbsp. freshly parsley chopped, and more for garnish

Instructions:

1. Melt one tbsp. Cook some butter in a large saucepan, then add oil. Season with salt and black pepper. Mahia, add, sauté. Cook for 5 minutes on each side. Transfer to a dish.

2. Apply one tbsp. of oil for the casserole. Cook for 4 minutes and add the spawn. Season with salt and pepper on a pan.

3. Heat butter to the skillet. Add garlic and pepper flakes and simmer until fragrant. Then add lemon zest, juice, and

Persil. Break the mahi-mahi into smaller pieces, then add asparagus and sauce.

4. Garnish before consuming.

Conclusions:

An important element to note is eating a great combination of lean meat, greens, and unprocessed carbs. The most efficient way to eat a balanced diet is simply adhering to whole foods, mainly because it is a healthy solution. It is crucial to understand that it is impossible to complete a ketogenic diet.

If you're a woman over 50, you may be far more interested in weight loss. Many women experience decreased metabolism at this age at a rate of about 50 calories per day. It can be incredibly hard to control weight gain by slowing the metabolism combined with less activity, muscle degradation and the potential for greater cravings. Many food options can help women over 50 lose weight and maintain healthy habits, but the keto diet has recently been one of the most popular.

CPSIA information can be obtained
at www.ICGtesting.com
Printed in the USA
BVHW041634120321
602399BV00009B/393